SOMETIMES AMAZING THINGS HAPPEN

HEARTBREAK AND HOPE ON THE BELLEVUE
HOSPITAL PSYCHIATRIC PRISON WARD

ELIZABETH FORD, MD

Regan Arts.
NEW YORK

Regan Arts.

65 Bleecker Street
New York, NY 10012

First Regan Arts hardcover edition, April 2017

Library of Congress Control Number: 2016932845

ISBN 978-1-941393-43-7

No one other than the author is identified by his or her real name in this book. Physical features and other potentially identifying characteristics also have been changed in many instances, and some characters and events are composites.

The views and opinions expressed in this book are solely those of the author. They are not and do not reflect the views or opinions of any organization or institution with which she is affiliated or has been affiliated or of anyone else employed by or affiliated with such organization or institution.

Interior design by Nancy Singer
Cover design by Richard Ljoenes

Printed in the United States of America

10 9 8 7 6 5 4 3 2 1

CONTENTS

CONTENTS

AUTHOR'S NOTE

The New York City jail system, with its hub on Rikers Island, manages approximately 1,000 people with serious mental illnesses on any given day, more than in all of the inpatient psychiatric units in the NYC public hospital system combined. While the volume is staggering and the implications for our society immense, the individual stories of these incarcerated men—who have been central to my experiences as a psychiatrist—are at once incredibly humbling, terrifying, and inspiring. Through them, I learned about survival and hope.

Like most jails, Rikers Island is primarily a detention center, a place originally intended to hold people charged with—not convicted of—crimes and considered too dangerous to be living in the community. For the eighty percent of detainees who are not serving a short misdemeanor sentence, the jail should be a quick stopover on the way from a judge's decision to retain them in custody to the decision to either release or transfer to prison. However, since the closure of many state psychiatric hospitals in the wake of the 1963 Community Mental Health Act and the escalation of the "war on drugs" in the 1980s, mental illness has been increasingly represented in the criminal justice system. The courts in New York City are overwhelmed, with long delays in case processing times. Rikers Island has become a jail where detainees stay for months, sometimes even years.

I wasn't aware of much of this when I began my internship at Bellevue Hospital in 2000 and had never given much thought to the island jail hidden in Flushing Bay. When I elected to do a month-long clinical rotation on Bellevue's 19th floor—a maximum-security hospital ward and the inpatient psychiatric unit for men at Rikers Island—I was quickly introduced to a world that was unlike any other. In only a few weeks, it was clear that being a doctor there was hard and confusing. One of my first patients, a cocaine addict with bipolar disorder, had "F.T.B." tattooed in scraggly block letters across his neck and scars all over his arms. I cringed when he proudly deciphered his neck for me as "Fuck the Bitch" and then melted when he showed me the cigarette burns from his mother and the self-inflicted razor cuts to his wrists from a recent suicide attempt. The many layers of complicated emotion underneath his violent body scars were both intriguing and scary.

This story describes my complicated and painful, yet sometimes incredibly joyful, journey into the world of psychiatry in jail. The seeds of this book began in 2007, in the eighth month of my second pregnancy, only days after I left my position as a psychiatrist on the Bellevue Hospital Prison Ward to start early maternity leave. At the time, my doctor had advised me to take it easy, not so much because of a specific physical risk but because my mental state was suffering. I was not sleeping well and I was constantly anxious and fearful. I started to write about my troubled thoughts and chaotic emotions as a way to download them from my brain—an attempt to get rid of them and, I hoped, make them less scary. The decision to publish some of those thoughts and stories was not made lightly. I am still deeply embedded in this work and have no interest in jeopardizing relationships or placing blame. I wish only to show this world through my own eyes, and in doing so, bring it a little more into the light.

For most doctors, working behind bars with patients whom others see as criminals, inmates, even "bodies," is not very appealing. The barriers to relieving suffering can be overwhelming and the rewards can seem few and far between. Yet, while the challenge has tested my spirit, my relationships with family and friends, and even my health, I feel lucky to have been given—and taken—the opportunity to learn and grow in an environment that brings out the best and the worst. I have come to see my success as a doctor not by how well I treat mental illness but by how well I respect and honor my patients' humanity, no matter where they are or what they have done.

The worlds described in this book—both the hospital and the jail it serves—are heartbreaking at times, infuriating at others, and always compelling. These worlds can easily shape the lives of patients, staff, or officers into hardened, angry, and traumatized versions of themselves. The characters in this book, including me, have all been exposed and transformed in various ways. While some of the stories involve behavior by clinical staff and officers that may seem callous, even cruel, every action and word should be seen in the context of the whole system—a complicated tangle of courts, jails, laws, unions, bureaucracy, and public opinion—that struggles to support the men and women tasked with caring for and keeping safe a population that many would like to forget. The simpler, sometimes inevitable, path for the staff is to absorb the chaos and culture, to decide that nothing can be done. The harder road is to fight, every day, to resist that transformation and find inspiration and hope in even the most dire situations.

The events described in this book take place from the year 2000 through 2014. I witnessed much progress during those years—progress that has more recently escalated at a rapid pace—at Bellevue, at Rikers Island, and in the city. However, many of the episodes that I recount here relate to complicated personal and professional situations that, from another's perspective, could be viewed differently. They are as I remember them and not the opinions of Bellevue Hospital, the City of New York Department of Correction, or any other agency or individual. I believe that the lives and health of the patients in this system will be diminished if their stories remain hidden.

To balance these considerations, and because my guiding principle as a physician is to "do no harm," I have changed the names of all of the characters except myself, and in many instances, I have changed physical features and other potentially identifying characteristics as well. Some individual staff members and patients depicted are actually composites of a few people who shared the same experiences. Conversations and dialogue are primarily reconstructed from memory, with only a few exceptions, and so are susceptible to the limits of my ability to recall those details. At the end of the day, I hope that I have succeeded in presenting these compelling narratives while also respecting my colleagues and, above all, my patients.

1

THE BODY BAG

At first, I don't realize that the rusty, unmarked metal gate on the corner of Twenty-sixth Street and First Avenue is the entryway to Bellevue, which looms over the East River on one side and the city's Poison Control Center on the other. Maybe the steady stream of people—amped-up, white-coated surgeons in scrubs, weary caregivers pushing invalids in wheelchairs, stumbling men who smell like alcohol and urine—should clue me in.

Since 1736, New York City has funded and supported Bellevue Hospital's mission of caring for anyone who walks in the door. It is the oldest public hospital in the country. Originally called a "Publick Workhouse and House of Correction," the modern-day hospital still treats patients who are mostly poor, uninsured, and homeless. Many are undocumented immigrants who speak no English. Some are under arrest. On the top floors sit the most famous psychiatric wards in the world. I know I am going to get to them someday, but first I have to learn to be a doctor.

Inside the gate, there is a decrepit garden with dying plants and dried-out fountains. A few weathered and lonely benches are scattered around. Perhaps this had once been a place of peace where you could quietly sit with a loved one, but now it is mostly a meet-up for drug dealers and their clients—and me. During the six months I spend working as an intern in medicine and neurology, I eat lunch on those benches, occasionally chatting with the addicts.

On my first day as a psychiatry intern, I happily join the rush of doctors and patients flowing into Bellevue. My fancy white coat with "NYU School of Medicine" stitched in purple cursive over the breast pocket is back at my apartment, hanging in a closet. Instead, I'm wearing my version of a fierce outfit—knee-high black boots with heels that bring me close to six feet tall, black tights, a short black skirt, a black sweater, and a thrift-store leather jacket that was a hand-me-up from my younger brother. The only clue that I'm a doctor is the stethoscope wrapped around my messenger bag. I am starting in the psychiatric emergency room to learn all about schizophrenia, antipsychotic medication, and how to commit someone to a hospital against his will.

Four narrow doors funnel people from the garden into a cavernous foyer with a set of brightly painted murals called "Materials for Relaxation," created in 1941 and newly restored. I push through the door on the far right to circumvent the bottleneck of people streaming into the "F" link, the central thoroughfare that leads from one end of the hospital complex to the other. I swerve to avoid a young woman pushing a stroller and pulling her crying toddler, only to bump into an elderly, inebriated black man stumbling over stained and torn pants that drag on the floor. The masses of people around us merely shift their path.

"I'm so sorry," I say, reaching to help steady the man. He grumbles incoherently and moves on.

The walls in the massive "F" link hallway are dull and white, decorated only by a handful of posters advertising insurance plans for low-income families and an upcoming Fourth of July garden picnic for the Bellevue staff.

I flash my NYU School of Medicine ID at the security guard manning the checkpoint for the hospital. I have just a few minutes before morning rounds start. I shove open a set of unmarked double doors on the ground floor, and I'm in the area of the hospital that only the really sick patients see: the back entrance to the ER, the emergency radiology suite, and the service elevators that move patients—including tiny, intubated preemie babies—up to the ICUs and inpatient suites. I know this world well from my medicine months, when I took care of people with heart attacks and diabetic comas. It is quieter back here than in the "F" link. The only people talking are the doctors and nurses; the patients and the transport techs who push their stretchers or wheelchairs are mostly silent.

I turn a corner, just before the hallway of X-ray rooms with their flashing red lights that signal radiation in progress, and look for the sign for CPEP, the Comprehensive Psychiatric Emergency Program.

"It's just past the station where the cops unload their weapons," Eileen, one of my co-residents, had told me on the phone the night before.

I see the sign, but from around another corner, I hear tense voices approaching.

"Hold him," one says. "It's just over there," says another.

I stop just in time to avoid the stretcher careening toward the CPEP. One EMS paramedic steers from the back while another stabilizes in front. Two NYPD cops walk on either side. They each have a hand on the body bag wiggling around on the stretcher.

"Hold still," one of the cops mutters to the bag. He looks across at his partner. "This ain't gonna be pretty."

Sounds of protest come from inside the bag—a muffled man's voice, deep and disturbed. He sounds like he's crying. The paramedics maneuver the stretcher into the doorway, jostling their passenger as they bump into a desk on the way in. I follow at a safe distance.

"Hold up," says a hospital police officer, holding his hand in front of my face. "You got to wait."

"But I work here," I protest, holding up my ID.

"Don't matter. You have to stay outside until this gets settled down." He closes the door in my face.

I try not to panic about being late for rounds on my first day and slump against the wall. I remember the first body bag I ever saw, the one that got me to medical school. I had been visiting Samantha, a close friend from high school and now a second-year medical student. One afternoon, she snuck me into the anatomy lab. The body bag was hidden inside one of many shiny dissection tables laid out in neat rows in the windowless, gymnasium-size room. I felt like I was in a stainless steel graveyard.

"You sure you want to see this?" Samantha asked. "It can be pretty gross if you're not used to it."

I wasn't sure. I gave her a quick nod anyway.

She went over to one of the covered tables and grabbed the handles on top of the hood. She struggled a bit to open it, but eventually the hood broke in two, each side hanging over the edge of the table. On the exposed flat surface lay a black body bag, zipped tight.

"Um . . . can we take a break?" I asked, starting to sweat.

"Sure, oh yeah, of course," she said as she laughed. "This was really hard for me the first time. Luckily, the students just started so they haven't dissected much. They've probably just cut into his back."

I turned away and dry-heaved.

"OK, I'm ready," I said, returning to the carcass and feeling both sick and exhilarated. Samantha slowly unzipped the bag. A waft of formalin and something kind of sweet hit me in the face. The top of a dead man's head came into view. I closed my eyes for a second and felt a little woozy. He was lying face down on the table. I assume he was a man, but in fact I saw nothing in this posterior view of an older, shriveled body to tell me for sure. His skin was pasty and a little yellow. He didn't have much hair covering his scalp, and folds of extra skin crowded around the back of his neck.

Samantha unzipped a bit more, and the cadaver's shoulders and upper back came into view. Flaps of skin from postmortem incisions had been restored as close to their original positions as possible. At some point soon, Samantha told me, the entire backside of this man—all of his muscles, nerves, blood vessels, and bones—would be inspected and dissected. He would then be flipped over, and the same would be done to his front side. Everything stayed inside the body bag, she explained, even the extra fat and skin that would need to be removed to dissect the internal organs. After the dissections were complete, the anatomy professors made sure that each body—likely to be cremated—contained all of the same stuff with which it started.

"Can you believe we get to do this?" Samantha asked.

"No," I answered quietly. I couldn't look away. He was not beautiful or warm, but he was inviting. My fingers were itching to pick up the scalpel lying by his side and cut into the flesh. I wanted desperately to understand what was going on inside his body. I wanted to know everything about this dead man.

"We should go," Samantha said.

She zipped the bag up and closed the steel hood. We scurried out of the room and into the cool, fresh hallway just as the security guard walked by.

"I have never seen anything like that," I said, awed by the power of that body. Surprising even myself, I whispered, "I think I'm going to medical school."

Now, seven years later and fifteen minutes after my arrival at the CPEP, the door opens up again and the officer ushers me in.

"Thanks," I say, quickly walking in and passing the EMS workers, one of whom has an empty body bag over his shoulder. I enter into an open space that has ten chairs bolted to the floor and borders a large windowed panel defining three separate sections of the CPEP. The first section, closest to the entrance and the hospital police officer, is where patients check in. Names and birthdates are confirmed, medical record numbers are assigned, and each new patient is logged into a giant ledger.

The next section is the triage room, which has 270-degree visibility. It's where a nurse does a preliminary interview and assesses whether a patient is stable enough to sit in the bolted chairs outside, or is so dangerous that he or she has to be locked in behind the door in the third section. Once inside this last area, no patient can get out without a doctor's order. For these patients, shoelaces and belts are removed to prevent hanging attempts, all property is taken and stored, and any illegal drugs are confiscated and flushed down the toilet.

There is a man handcuffed to a stretcher next to the triage room, asleep. He has a few bruises on his face, and his clothes are torn and dirty. His twisted body and sprawled legs give him the unnatural appearance of someone who has been medically induced into sleep. The cops I saw in the hallway are sitting in the chairs watching him. They look uneasy.

One of the nurses lets me in through a locked door into the triage room, grumbling about how "those interns really need to get their own keys." I scoot past her and head to where the doctors, medical students, and social workers are already gathered and talking about their patients.

"Sorry," I whisper as I sit down in the last available folding chair.

"Nice of you to join us," the attending psychiatrist, Dr. Leon, says to me.

"I was stuck in the hallway for about fifteen minutes," I say defensively. "The officer wouldn't let me in."

"Oh yeah," says Dr. Leon, softening. "That was the NYPD case. Spitting and fighting. We had to 5 and 2 him." Although I am new to psychiatry I've already heard these numbers on the medicine and neurology wards referring to 5 mg of Haldol and 2 mg of Ativan, a typical cocktail of intramuscular medications given to patients who are aggressively agitated. "Should be awake in a few hours, and then we can get him out of here."

I am too new and too afraid to ask what I am thinking: *What if he needs to be in the hospital?* I listen to the rest of the report and notice that Dr. Leon assigns himself the NYPD case; the patient's name is James. Patients like James get brought in for all kinds of reasons—from requesting Ritalin to trying to hang themselves in the precinct house. The cops know that they could be sued—or fired—if someone in their custody is denied medical or psychiatric care, even if the request is for a pill that the "perp" hasn't taken for 20 years. Most of the doctors don't want to assess the NYPD patients; there are so many of them, thousands per year, and only a very small percentage get admitted to the hospital. Dr. Leon is trying to keep his psychiatrists happy by picking up the case. I ask if I can tag along.

Hours later, close to the end of the shift, we go to see James. He is still groggy from the medication but alert enough to answer questions. He's been charged with second-degree assault, the cops say, because he punched a stranger on the subway. I listen to Dr. Leon ask James a rapid-fire set of standard questions.

"How come the cops brought you to the hospital?"

"Don't ask me," James replies gruffly.

"Do you take psych meds?"

"Someone gave me some of those once, but I don't take 'em. Don't need 'em."

"Ever been in the hospital before?"

"Check the record, man. I been here a hundred times before."

"Are you suicidal?"

"No."

"Do you want to hurt anyone else?"

"Just those cops who roughed me up."

"Are you hearing voices?"

James laughs. "Just yours."

A few other basic questions follow, and Dr. Leon and I return to the doctors' area. We don't have James's medical record to see if he's been admitted or evaluated here before—this was in the days before computerized medical records.

"This is the form you have to fill out to give to the cops for arraignment," says Dr. Leon. I have no idea what "arraignment" means, so Dr.

Leon gives me a doctor's explanation: it is the hearing where James sees a judge for the first time and gets an attorney. The form says that James has been "psychiatrically cleared for arraignment" and doesn't need to be admitted to the hospital.

"How do you decide if he's OK for arraignment?" I ask.

"It's a really low threshold—basically, whether he can stand up in front of the judge and whether he can keep from hurting himself or anyone else in the courtroom."

I am too naive to know that this is just a CPEP definition that evolved because there is no legal definition of "stable for arraignment." I watch as Dr. Leon hands the paperwork to the cops, tells them James can go, and heads to the next patient on the list. I think about the way James presented—arrested for a stranger attack—and the need for a body bag and heavy tranquilizers to calm him down, the short, clipped answers about medication and hospitalizations. There is more happening with James than the quick assessment revealed. But after he heads out the CPEP door to the waiting NYPD squad car, I never see him again.

2

CAUGHT BETWEEN THE CRACKS

After a few months of facing extreme cases in the CPEP—*was this woman going to kill herself if I discharged her? Was the paranoid homeless man going to punch me when I told him that he was staying in the hospital?*—I finish that assignment and, after a weekend to recover, head to my next clinical rotation.

On my way to the upstairs inpatient psychiatry units Monday morning, I find myself squished into the back corner of the hospital's express elevator. A pharmacy technician carrying a few bags of saline, and a drug sales rep in high heels and tailored suit are on either side of me. There are a few white-coated medical students talking loudly about their last quiz, but the rest of us are silent, staring at the illuminated floor numbers as we make our way up. I close my eyes and take some slow, deep breaths, trying to be patient as the elevator gradually empties at each stop.

I get off at the nineteenth floor. To the left, just past the "Notice of Patient Rights" posted in the hallway, a set of closed yellow double doors signals the beginning of 19 North, the psychiatry inpatient unit at Bellevue where all the new NYU psychiatry residents learn how to take care of patients with serious mental illnesses. These are not the patients who come into the CPEP intoxicated on cocaine or alcohol, sleep it off

9

for a few hours, and then walk back out onto First Avenue. The patients on 19 North have done things like lock themselves in their rooms for weeks to avoid an alien invasion, try to commit suicide by jumping from the Brooklyn Bridge, or firmly believe that they are God.

Just before the double doors, a large white sign with a left arrow indicates the Bellevue Hospital Prison Ward. I know a little bit about this place from the CPEP—this is where James would have gone if Dr. Leon had admitted him. The rumors about the prison ward—that it is dangerous, creepy, and full of psychopathic killers like Hannibal Lecter—are scary and intriguing, but I don't believe that a ward full of patients like James can be that bad. Right now, all I can see is a freight elevator, a set of scuffed blue lockers, and another set of yellow doors opening into an office suite. It looks just like anywhere else in the hospital.

A tiny Filipino woman with a giant smile approaches me as I'm staring at the white sign.

"Come in, come in," she says cheerfully, introducing herself as May and guiding me toward 19 North.

I reach out for a handshake, but she is already ahead of me, motioning for me to follow. I am quickly escorted into an office and directed to put my coat and bag on the chair inside. Then May leads me through a warren of rooms and hallways to an unmarked, locked white door.

"Rounds are just about to start," says May as she pulls a ring of keys from her pocket. "Just go through this door, turn right, and the conference room is past the nursing station. The other residents are all in there."

She ushers me through and is gone. I stand alone in a very long hallway already busy with activity. Someone who looks like a patient with loose-fitting clothes, knotted hair, and a stooped posture is on the pay phone a few feet away, whispering into the handset. A round, short woman with a hospital ID tells a patient to get back into his room. Two patients—a young Hispanic woman in a rumpled T-shirt and pajama pants and a tall black man in jeans—are pacing up and down the hallway. He speaks to her in a very loud and animated manner; she has a blank stare on her face. A woman with braids piled on top of her head and light brown scrubs sits in front of a room at the far end of the hallway. She is holding a clipboard in her lap with her chin resting heavily on her chest. In the middle of it all, the nursing station juts into the hallway of the unit like a glass-paneled observatory.

When I enter the conference room, there are only two seats left at the giant square table. One is next to Dr. Miller, the head psychiatrist, or unit chief, for 19 North. I pick the other available seat, next to Eileen.

"Hey," I whisper. "Am I really late?"

"No," Eileen reassures me. "I think we're just waiting for the chief resident."

In the world of academic medical training, there is a very clear hierarchy. Medical students are at the bottom. Just above them are interns, like me, newly graduated doctors who may or may not have an actual license to practice medicine. Then come the second-, third-, and maybe fourth- or fifth-year residents. Psychiatry is a four-year residency.

After the residents come the chief residents, in their last year of training and selected to help organize and lead the residency program. Finally, when the residency is all over and a doctor no longer needs formal guidance, he or she becomes an attending physician. Attendings do not have to get supervision for medical decisions and are the "doctors of record" in teaching hospitals like Bellevue. Dr. Miller is the top attending on 19 North. He has the reputation for being brilliant and demanding.

Suddenly, a whirlwind of a man comes through the door on the opposite side of the conference room. It's the chief resident, Marc, who has John Lennon glasses and shoulder-length blond hair and is wearing a brown leather coat and a striped bow tie. He'd caught my eye across the bar at a "welcome to residency" gathering eight months before, but I hadn't seen him since.

"Sorry, sorry," he says as he quickly scans the room, then glances at the patient list waiting for him at the table. "Let's get started."

Marc runs down the list of the twenty-five current patients, stopping for discussion whenever someone has an update or concern about a patient's condition. Despite my first-day jitters, I boldly make coy eye contact with Marc whenever I can.

"What's the deal with Mary?" asks Dr. Miller. "She's been here for six weeks. Why is she still in the hospital?"

Mary is a sixty-eight-year-old widow with children (and, now, grandchildren) whom she left behind in South Carolina when she took a Greyhound bus up to New York forty years before, as her schizophrenia was starting to get really bad. She hasn't been in touch with her family since. Age and illness, including high blood pressure and diabetes, have turned her life into a revolving door of shelters, hospitals, and group homes.

"We're waiting for the nursing home to come and interview her," says Carolyn, a social worker who moonlights as a musician. "They don't want to take someone with schizophrenia," she continues, "but I'll keep calling. They have to at least talk . . ."

"I'm not going to wait much longer," interrupts Dr. Miller. "There are patients who need her bed more than she does. She can't stay here forever."

"I'll work on it."

"Great," says Marc, breaking the tension with his upbeat tone. He moves us along and begins randomly assigning several patients to each of the interns. I get Mary.

I spend the next few days getting to know my patients, talking to them in the shared dining room of the unit or while pacing back and forth along the fifty yards of the hallway. Mary prefers to pace, but we don't go very fast; she shuffles along and rests her arm on mine. She is deeply stubborn about her independence and does not believe there is anything wrong with her mind. She attributes her many psychosis-induced hospitalizations to "bad luck." She sometimes talks about her family back in South Carolina, but describes them as if they were characters in a book, rather than her own relatives.

I get impatient with Mary; not only do I not have time for leisurely walks, but I feel completely useless as she avoids every question related to her illness.

"Oh, that's nothing," she says. "Nothing for you to worry about."

"But I'm your doctor," I protest. "It's my job to worry about you."

"Let me worry about myself," she snaps.

I am silenced by her anger and go back to making small talk about the weather and her diabetes. I see why Dr. Miller thinks she should go.

It's a relief when I get to pick up a new patient the next day. Patients are admitted to 19 North at all hours from the CPEP, but we only do new-admission interviews after rounds each morning. Any patients admitted later than that are "eyeballed" by an intern to make sure anything urgent, like a suicide watch, is started immediately.

Dr. Miller has specific requirements about these interviews. They are done in front of the team—everyone needs to see, hear, and sometimes smell the same things. No looking at the medical chart in advance. No note-taking. No asking for help from the team unless you are ready to give up the interview. And you must establish the basics before getting into any symptoms. This is my first time doing one of these interviews.

My palms are sweaty as I offer my new patient a chair at the table and sit down a few feet away. The team is seated around us with their pens poised.

"Good morning, Diane. I'm Dr. Ford," I say, proffering my hand.

"Hi." She takes my hand weakly and then drops her own back into her lap.

"This is your team," I say, gesturing behind me. "We'd like to find out how you came to the hospital and how we can help you."

She keeps her eyes down and nods. A bald spot on the top of her head reveals a pink scar surrounded by new peach fuzz. The rest of her curly black hair obscures her face. She is wearing a loose pink sweatshirt and no bra, her large breasts resting on the waistband of her slacks.

"Diane, how old are you?" I am supposed to ask first about her demographic information—age, education, housing status.

"Fifty-two."

"Where are you living?"

"I have a space," she says. "It's not always the same, but Robert and I are together, and that's all that matters."

"Who's *Robert?*" I ask. I'm not sticking to the script.

"My fiancé. He's wonderful. He stays with me all the time. He sleeps in the garden outside when I'm in the hospital. He's probably there now."

"How long have you been with *Robert?*"

"Diane where do you live exactly?" interrupts Dr. Miller, and that ends my interview. I can no longer ask any more questions because I have deviated from the script. I sit in silence, shame, and anger. I lasted only four questions. And now Eileen, Marc, my fellow interns, Dr. Miller—and, most importantly, Diane—are going to think I am an incompetent doctor. I hold back my tears.

Diane looks up at the new voice asking questions and repeats the answers she gave to me. Dr. Miller eventually gets all the information we need. Her scar is a remnant from a recent tumor resection—a meningioma that had grown large on the surface of her brain. She was paranoid prior to the tumor and had been in and out of psychiatric hospitals, but now she is also hallucinating. She hears harsh voices yelling at her throughout the night, chastising her for being too fat, too crazy, too old. She doesn't take her medicine because of a combination of fear that she is being poisoned and some memory loss after the surgery. I try to pay attention to the other details of her story, but the still-thumping blood in my ears keeps me focused instead on Dr. Miller.

As soon as the interview is over, I scurry into my tiny office. I sit there and try, with some effort, to breathe slowly. I pull my copy of

Essentials of Psychopharmacology from a shelf and look up ziprasidone, the new antipsychotic medication that we are going to start for Diane. I again try to focus my attention on my patient, but cannot get Dr. Miller out of my mind. I have to do something about it.

I leave my office, hold my head high, and walk to the end of the office suite. Dr. Miller's door is slightly ajar.

"Excuse me, Dr. Miller." I say. "Can I talk to you for a second?"

"Of course, come in," he says. "Sit down."

I look for a seat in his small office and find only the analytic couch he has managed to fit against one wall. I sit down on the edge, careful not to recline.

"I . . . I . . ." I start cautiously. "I want to talk to you about the interview with Diane."

"Yes?"

"I really didn't think it was fair the way you interrupted me so quickly." My words spill out fast. "I know you have a particular way you like to teach interns to interview, but why didn't you even give me a chance? I mean, four questions? How am I going to learn anything that way?"

Dr. Miller listens as I speak, leaning back in his swivel chair and crossing his fingers in front of him.

"Do you understand what I'm saying?" I ask louder. "Does this make any sense?" Frustrated by his silence and my rage, I am crying. My tears embarrass me.

"I do," he slowly responds, offering me a box of tissues. "And I think you are being too hard on yourself. The first interview is always the most difficult. You've been here, what, five days? By the time your four months here are finished, you will be able to do an amazing first interview. That's what I'm trying to teach you." His words and tone are not unkind, but I am not satisfied.

"Why do I have to do it your way? Does it really matter, as long as I get the information?"

Dr. Miller cracks a smile. "You are persistent, aren't you?"

"Yes. And I'm going to continue to be that way." I start to laugh softly, realizing how much I sound like a petulant child. "Sorry. I just don't think the way you cut me off was fair."

"Hmmm," sighs Dr. Miller, giving me no indication of whether he agrees with me or not. After a few seconds of uncomfortable silence, he concludes, "I think you and I are going to get along just fine." I leave his office not sure of whether I totally agree with him, but feeling better than when I went in.

Over the next month, I get to know Robert, Diane's fiancé, better than Diane. I spend part of each day on 19 North sitting on the floor in Diane's room while she lies in her bed with her face to the wall. Mostly, I wait in silence for ten minutes to see if she feels like sharing. At first, I had tried sitting in a chair, then resting against a back wall, but both positions were too threatening to her. She only speaks, however briefly, when I am on the floor.

Robert, however, I see two to three times a week in the garden when I'm eating lunch. He tells me stories of Diane—her wish to be held each night while they try to sleep on the shabby mattress in their tiny one-room apartment, her infectious laugh, her struggle to keep her girlish figure on so many medications—and I slowly get to know her through him. He stays in that garden from the time the gates open at 6:00 a.m. until visiting hours on the unit at 2:00 p.m. Sometimes, Diane refuses to see him—a sign of the severity of her illness—but Robert comes anyway. When the nurse tells him that time's up, he heads back to the mattress and waits for the next day.

I think of Mary and her lost family in South Carolina sometimes when I am talking to Diane. Mary does not have a Robert in her life. She doesn't have someone to take her home once she leaves the hospital. Even though Dr. Miller is right about Mary—she is no longer acutely dangerous—everyone on the unit knows that she will stop her medicine the moment she is discharged and will end up back at Bellevue—or worse, at the morgue. After a few days off of her antipsychotic meds, she will get paranoid about her blood pressure pills and stop them. Then she will start talking to strangers in the subway and riding the trains back and forth until one of the conductors insists that she leave. She will probably forget to eat.

So Carolyn, the musical social worker, continues her efforts to find a nursing home for Mary. Every week, Dr. Miller reminds us exactly how many days Mary has been in the hospital—80, then 94, and now we're up to 108. Mary has had a few interviews with nursing homes, but none of them are a fit. Two of the nursing homes say they can't manage her level of mental illness, and the other requires that Mary have a room-mate. Mary insists on her privacy and refuses to go.

"She's driving up our length of stay," Dr. Miller says in rounds. "Dr. Ford, are you doing anything with her medicine?"

"No," I reply cautiously. "She doesn't have side effects and she seems better." I look for support from Marc, with whom I have developed a flirtatious friendship, but he is distracted by paperwork.

"Is she still dangerous?" Dr. Miller asks.

"Uh, no, not really, but . . ."

He turns to Carolyn and interrupts my answer with a question for her. "Have you found any place that will take Mary?"

"Yes," she responds, as cautious as I am. "But Mary doesn't want to go there."

"I don't really care where Mary wants to go at this point," fumes Dr. Miller. "She does not need to be in the hospital; she is taking up a bed for someone who does, and we aren't providing any real treatment for her. She needs to leave this week."

"Wait," I say from across the table. "We can't send her out yet. She won't make it. Please let us keep trying!"

"Dr. Ford, I have given you ample time to keep trying. We would all like to keep every patient in the hospital until there is a perfect plan on the outside, but that's just not how it works anymore. Mary wants to leave the hospital, and if she wants to go to a shelter instead of a nursing home, that's her choice. But she has to leave this unit. Please start working on her discharge summary and prescriptions."

"No!" I yell, slapping my open hand on the rounds table with a *thwap* that is all anger and defiance.

Eileen and the other residents are shocked. Carolyn is sitting halfway between Dr. Miller and me, and can't figure out which way to look. She sinks lower into her chair. Marc looks up, stunned.

"Excuse me?" asks Dr. Miller as if saying, "Do you want to fail this rotation?" I don't think he is used to this kind of resistance.

"I'm sorry, Dr. Miller," I stammer, red-faced yet firm in my conviction. "I can't discharge Mary. It's not safe. I know she wants to go, but I just can't do it. We will find a place for her, I promise."

"That is not acceptable," is his icy reply. "She is perfectly safe, and we cannot hold her against her will unless she is dangerous. We do not babysit patients. Carolyn, please help Dr. Ford get Mary ready for discharge."

I don't hear what Carolyn says because the throbbing of blood in my ears is so loud. After a few moments, I whisper, "I won't do it, Dr. Miller. With all due respect, if you want her discharged you will have to sign the papers yourself." My tone does not match the strength of the words but the point gets across.

"Fine, let's talk about this later," says Dr. Miller. And with that, rounds are over.

I wait day after day to receive my punishment, while Carolyn works tirelessly to find a place for Mary to go. Dr. Miller and I have difficulty making eye contact during rounds, but he is civil and professional. Mary gets another nursing home interview a week later. This time, it's a fit.

On the morning of her departure, before rounds, I shake her hand and wish her luck. Her eyes look distant; I'm not sure she even understands where she is going. When Dr. Miller crosses her off the patient list and smiles at me with a sigh of relief—and maybe, possibly, a hint of respect—I know the fight was worth it.

3

STARS OVER BELLEVUE

It's just after 11:00 p.m. on Valentine's Day, almost two years later. I'd spent one year rotating on inpatient units at NYU's various training hospitals, and the following year learning how to treat outpatients in a clinic. Tonight, I am back where I feel most comfortable, the wards of Bellevue's "H" building. The twenty-three-story hospital was completed in 1986 and the top floors house most of the inpatient psychiatry units formerly located in the aging Bellevue Psychiatric Hospital, now a men's shelter, a few blocks north.

In eight hours, the day shift will come on duty, and the place will be frenetic, dirty, and loud again, but for now, it's almost peaceful. Midway into my third year of residency and spending most of my day with stable outpatients, I moonlight every Friday night as the only doctor on the twelve psychiatric units, mostly on the eighteenth through twentieth floors. I need the money to help pay back my student loans, but that's not the only reason I work these shifts. I crave the excitement and the volatility of the overnights. On Friday nights, I really feel like a doctor.

The first few hours of every shift are predictable: 19 North will call first with a list of simple orders that the interns forgot to write during the day. There'll be a diet order change to "low sodium" for a patient with newly diagnosed high blood pressure, or a Benadryl order to help

19

someone sleep. The detox unit, 20 South, houses patients who need to safely sober up and, with any luck, move on to more long-term rehab programs; the unit nurse will call next about a handful of patients who wish to sign out AMA (against medical advice). I have to make sure the patients know all the risks of leaving early.

"You know that you can get seizures or heart problems, or possibly even die, from alcohol withdrawal?" I tell one of them. "Are you sure you don't want to stay a few more days so we can get you into some real treatment?"

"Naw, I'm good," is a common reply. "I'll just grab another drink when I get out. That will stop the shakes."

The calls around 11:00 p.m. for sleep medication signal about an hour to go before the Department of Correction (DOC) intake pens on the nineteenth floor start jumping. I grab some M&M's and a Diet Pepsi from a vending machine and head to 19 West, the psychiatry inpatient unit on the hospital's "prison ward." It's imprecisely named, because it's actually a jail, a detention facility for defendants awaiting trial or those sentenced to relatively short periods of incarceration for misdemeanor offenses. In the 1980s, half of the nineteenth floor was turned into a maximum security outpost of the massive New York City jail system, fourteen separate jails that are spread out across the five boroughs. Nine jails are located on a 415-acre island in Flushing Bay, 100 yards west of LaGuardia Airport, called Rikers Island. The unit at Bellevue, including 19 West, is for male inmates who need hospitalization. Facilities in downtown Manhattan, the Bronx, Brooklyn, and a psychiatric unit for women at Elmhurst Hospital in Queens round out the fourteen.

I know 19 West well. It is not so different from the other psychiatric units; it has a full complement of nursing staff, social workers, psychiatrists, psychologists, nursing techs, and activity and art therapists. Hospital specialists, like orthopedic surgeons and infectious disease specialists, are available as needed. All the clinical staff, from the housekeepers to the psychiatrists, work for Bellevue or NYU. They are not part of the DOC and do not report to or take orders from the officers, except around issues related directly to security.

The patients—mostly poor Blacks or Hispanics in their twenties and thirties with serious mental illnesses—are similar to the patients on the other psychiatry floors, with two notable exceptions. All of the patients on 19 West are men, and they are all in jail.

In 2003, the New York City jail system took care of about 14,000 inmates on any given day (though by 2015, the number had dropped to approximately 10,000 inmates a day). Bellevue sees only the tiny fraction of inmates suffering from such severe illness that they need hospitalization. Very few of them have been sentenced for a crime; most have not been convicted and are waiting for a plea deal or trial. Some cannot even pay a one-dollar bail.

I've already received six messages from 19 West for requests like renewing medication that will expire the next day or for a different breakfast order for the morning. Unless it's an emergency, I try to hold all the 19 West calls until everything else is done. I only want to go in and out of the jail gates once.

Connecting the entrances to 19 North and 19 West is a wide corridor lined on both sides by service elevators. The ones on the east side carry freight—patients on gurneys, medications, construction supplies. The west elevator across the hall is massive. I've never been in that one—I've never even seen the inside, just two wide, unpolished doors of stainless steel. Patients in the jail system come up and go down on that elevator. No one who isn't in cuffs or wearing a uniform ever gets in.

The corridor dead-ends at a sally port past an old and unused airport-style metal detector and a small dingy waiting area with dented visitor lockers, a broken TV, and a Pepsi machine with a sign warning "Use at your own risk." Enormous metal gates made out of jail bars, painted white and peeling, guard the entrance.

At the sally port, I see the officer standing in the control room on the other side of the first gate, looking at the closed circuit monitors above his head. The monitors are linked to live feeds from 19 West and 19 South, the jail's medical-surgical unit down the hall. Part of the officer's job is to open the gate for me, but his eyes are fixed on something on the screens. I wait a few seconds longer and read over the now-familiar signs warning me that assaulting a correction officer is a felony punishable by up to seven years in prison, and that visitors will be subject to prosecution if they bring any kind of contraband into the unit. Listed along with knives, guns, and narcotics are electronic devices and pagers. I've got an old-school digital pager clipped to my belt, but no one has ever stopped me for it.

"On the gate," I finally yell to get the officer's attention.

The electric gate creaks and groans and slowly moves along its track. I slip through as soon as I can, then wait for it to reach its limit and reverse, sliding shut. It goes much faster closing. I had gotten my shoulder clipped by the gate the previous week. In this anteroom of sorts, there is a weapons unloading station. Two waist-high metal boxes with wire mesh covering the openings at the top and raised sides rising almost to shoulder level to shield in case of a stray bullet.

The officer checks my ID—he's new and not the regular guy who usually just waves me through—and then pushes a button to open the next gate. The 19 West unit has earned the nickname "the Wild West," because the most dangerous patients in the hospital are admitted here. These are men who have just tried to kill themselves, have just tried to kill someone else, or are too psychotic to survive in jail. Although there are mental health clinics in each facility and, in some, housing units specifically for those with serious illness, it is hard to stay safe at Rikers Island. As best I can tell from the patients—my only source of information, as I have yet to visit the Island myself—it's more like a war zone full of mistrust and unpredictable dangers. Many of the patients arrive at Bellevue with fresh bruises and fractures that go unexplained.

Nineteen West is guarded by another heavy gate that has to be opened with a giant old-fashioned key. The "A" post officer, a fifty-something-year-old named Monique, whose uniform pulls tight around her hips and who is biding her time until she can retire in a year with a full pension, controls everyone going in and out of the unit. At this time of night, it's easy to get in the unit. Monique knows that once I arrive, the sleep meds will get ordered so the nurses can hand them out.

"Welcome, Doc," she says with a weary smile. "I hope you can calm things down in there."

Within ten seconds of walking into the long, wide 19 West hallway, I see Pedro, a twenty-five-year-old member of the Latin Kings gang, walk up to the nursing station window near the entrance in his hospital pajamas, lower himself onto the tile floor, and start wildly thrashing around. Anne, the nurse who picks up extra shifts as I do on Friday nights, comes charging out of the nursing station. Then several correction officers who are assigned posts on the unit start heading in Pedro's direction.

"Dr. Ford!" Anne exclaims. "You've got to do something about him! He's been acting like this all night. Didn't you get any of my pages?"

I look at my pager and sheepishly shrug my shoulders when I see that Anne has indeed paged me multiple times.

"I can't keep interrupting everything to deal with his problems," she goes on. "Do you know all the work I have to do? The evening shift, what did they do? Nothing. Leave me all of the admission paperwork and notes to write. Look at this, I have . . ."

Anne's a chronically frazzled nurse, and as she rattles on about her night, I grow impatient.

"Hey, Anne," I interrupt her. "I hear you. But what about Pedro?"

"See for yourself," she grunts, motioning in his direction.

Pedro is still moving around on the floor, his eyes and jaw clenched tight. I can tell from the very deliberate shakes of his limbs that he is not having a real seizure. His pajama pants are wet; I'm pretty sure he poured water on himself to make it look like he had urinated.

"Pedro, come on, open your eyes," I say.

He keeps his eyes closed and whimpers about having a seizure. His legs stop shaking, but his right hand keeps flapping around.

I kneel next to him.

"Pedro, I'm going to touch your hand, OK?"

Pedro's right hand keeps moving as I hold his wrist and check his pulse. I don't expect to feel anything unusual; I just want to see what he will do. We hold hands like that for about thirty seconds while two nursing techs I hadn't seen before lean against the wall and roll their eyes. The techs are the ones who spend the most time with the patients, checking on everyone at least every half hour, handing out meal trays, watching TV, playing Ping-Pong in the rec room, and sometimes staying with a patient around the clock to make sure he doesn't kill himself. Although these patients are in jail, they are free to wander around the unit.

"Please, this is ridiculous," says Anne. Pedro eventually stops moving his hand.

"Great news," I say to his still-closed eyes. "It looks like you didn't have a seizure. But what just happened there? I don't really understand."

He pops open his eyes and glares at me.

"I just had a seizure, Doc!" he yells. "What, you blind?"

"Um, no," I answer, distracted for a second by a new number coming in on my pager. I turn back to Pedro.

"How do you know it was a seizure?"

"I was lying there, shaking on the ground, for Christ's sake. Didn't you see that? It was right in front of the window."

"So you remember it?" I ask. He knows that I've caught him. Seizures like he's describing almost always involve a loss of consciousness and memory.

"No, not really," he backtracks, thinking about how to change his answer. "I just figured, since I was here at the window, that it must have happened here. I need some Ativan for it, at least two milligrams."

"He's not getting any Ativan!" Anne bellows from the nursing station. "He's just a drug seeker!"

"Hold on," I say impatiently to both Pedro and Anne.

I go into the nursing station and pick up the desk phone to return the page. It's the nineteenth-floor intake area where all the jail patients get processed in and out of the units. They get stripped, searched, ID'd, and put in one of several holding pens. Officer Maddox works in intake most Friday nights. Last Friday, he gave me a pint of milk and two small boxes of Kellogg's Corn Pops left over from one of the patient trays when he heard my stomach growling at 3:00 a.m.

"Doc, we got three for you, including Reynaldo," Officer Maddox tells me over the phone, referring to the patients I have to evaluate before the night is up. "He bangs his head a lot, but he's asleep right now," says Maddox, who apparently has seen Reynaldo before. "I got the paperwork for you in intake."

"Are they OK to sit there for a bit?" I ask. "I've got a thing happening on 19 West." I look over my shoulder at Pedro.

"Yeah, for a little while. I don't know the other two, but they seem OK for now. Just get here when you can."

The bus from Rikers Island must have arrived while I was with Pedro. It's a tricked-out white school bus with "Corrections" painted in bold blue letters along the sides and steel mesh covering all the windows. Only nine miles separate the Island from the hospital, but I frequently hear that the bus ride can take six to ten hours—"bus therapy" as the patients and a few doctors say sardonically. The psychiatrists at the jail are so inundated with the thousands of mentally ill people locked up there that they can't watch everyone closely.

And most of the patients—except the women and adolescents, who have their own jails—move around from facility to facility in what seems like a DOC shell game. Patients are moved after a fight, because of gang affiliations, or because they need treatment that's only offered in a different jail. Sometimes it seems as though they're moved just to keep them from getting too comfortable. Each transfer can mean days spent in the intake pens at the sending and receiving facilities, even if the next location is the building next door. The psychiatrists work hard just to make sure the patients get seen at all.

The Friday night bus usually carries the patients who the officers on Rikers Island are worried won't make it through the weekend. These are the ones found hanging in a cell and cut down just before they die. Or patients who have languished for days until some diligent officer notices—once the chaos of the week has died down—that, in their psychosis, they have begun to eat their own feces instead of their meals. Or those who are so delusional that they listen to the voices in their heads telling them to cut off a limb in order to save their souls. DOC will refer these patients to the on-call psychiatrist at Rikers, who expedites the order to transfer them to Bellevue.

Once they get to the back entrance of the hospital, the patients are shackled together in their orange DOC jumpsuits and shuffled through multiple security checkpoints before heading onto the giant steel elevator. Officers with unloaded weapons walk on either side of this chain gang.

All sorts of patients arrive in the intake area. Men like Reynaldo. Or like Lisa, a pre-op transgender woman who is constantly on protective watch and followed by an officer with a camera to make sure nothing "suspicious" happens. She lives as a woman but is kept with all the men because she still has a penis.

Then there is Silvio, a man accused of five counts of murder, who's apparently in the Mafia. Every Friday, he makes some small cuts on his wrists with a newly acquired piece of floor tile or a sharpened battery casing, and tells the overwhelmed psychiatrist at Rikers Island that he's suicidal. What he doesn't say is that it's easier for his mother to visit him at Bellevue on Saturday instead of taking two subways and a bus to the Island. This "cut-and-switch" usually gets him a weekend admission, just enough for his mom to bring him some magazines and an update about the family business. I could refuse to admit him, but once, a couple of months before, another doctor sent him back, and he returned eight hours later with a ten-inch slice to his upper thigh that required a trip to the ICU. It's safer and easier to give him a bed for a few nights and be done with it.

"Thanks," I sigh to Officer Maddox. Silvio and Lisa aren't on the bus tonight—Silvio was transferred to prison a few days before, and I guess Lisa didn't make the DOC transfer list. "Page me if something changes," I say before hanging up the phone.

I turn back to Pedro, still scowling at me from the floor. I force my face into a calm smile.

"Let's figure out what's going on, Pedro. Are you in pain?" I ask.

"I just had a seizure!" he bellows again.

I put my palms out in frustration and helplessness, resisting the urge to put them on my hips and roll my eyes.

"I can't help you if I don't have more information. How about you go back to your bed and rest and I'll check the chart for your orders?"

"I'm staying right here . . ." he starts just as I see something more important out of the corner of my eye. An older patient who's been pacing the halls is suddenly down.

"OK, stay there," I yell over my shoulder to Pedro as I race down the hall with the two aides. We find the patient, a middle-aged white man named Bill, on the floor biting his tongue and shaking.

"Two milligrams of Ativan!" I shout down the hallway to Anne.

The aides and I roll Bill on his side and stare uncomfortably as he jerks and clenches and labors with his breathing. After less than a minute, he stops shaking.

"Watch him," I say to the aides, and hurry back to the nursing station and the phone, skirting Pedro, who's still camped out on the floor. Anne is in the medication room, a tiny closet of a space attached to the nursing station. It has a locked sliding door, a double-locked cabinet containing the narcotics—including Ativan—and a red plastic sharps bucket for used needles.

I find the chart for Bill and call the medicine consult, a third-year resident who manages all the admissions and transfers to the medicine beds on the sixteenth and seventeenth floors. He answers as though he hasn't slept in 24 hours.

"What's the emergency?" he barks.

"A patient up here just had a seizure," I say.

"Is he still seizing?"

"No. But he just came in from Rikers Island this morning and we don't have any labs on him. Looks like he hasn't been talking today, just pacing around."

His chart is not that helpful. The Rikers psychiatrist who sent Bill to the hospital wrote NEEDS ADMISSION in caps across the referral form, but neglected to include necessary information like Bill's age, his medical history, or even why he needed psychiatric care.

"Get some labs, load him with Dilantin, and someone will come see him in the morning," says the consult.

"I'm worried about him," I reply. "Can you come up and see him sooner?"

I hear a grunt on the other end.

"Yeah, OK," comes the reluctant response. "Where is he?"

"19 West."

A pause. "Oh. I can't get up there tonight. He's going to have to wait until the morning. It doesn't sound that serious anyway. One seizure is probably not something to worry about."

"Wait, what do you mean you can't get up here?" I demand, before realizing what has just happened. He doesn't want to come in the jail unit. If I push too hard, the consult won't want to help me either, and Bill won't get seen before the morning.

"How about I call you when the blood results are back?" I offer as an alternative.

"Yeah, that's good. Give me his name and medical record number. I'll put him on my list."

After we hang up, I stand still for a moment, feeling dejected.

"You still want me to give him the Ativan?" hollers Anne from the medication room, holding the loaded syringe.

"No, he's stopped seizing," I tell her.

"I haven't stopped seizing!" shouts Pedro through the open nursing station window. "I need the Ativan!"

"Pedro, we're not talking about you," I snap. "You are welcome to go back to your bedroom, but I've got to deal with another patient right now."

I turn back to Anne.

"I'm going to get his blood, and as soon as we can, we'll give him some Dilantin. I'll put the orders in."

Anne mutters about how she drew up the Ativan for nothing.

"Can I get some butterflies from in there?" I ask, referring to the tiny gauge needles I'll need to draw Bill's blood. The plastic grips at the end of the needles look like butterfly wings. They are kept in the medication room in a drawer under the narcotics closet along with gauze, alcohol pads, and bandages. Anne grumbles while she gets me the supplies.

Bill's veins are squishy through his skin and roll under my fingers, but the butterfly goes in smoothly, and the thick, dark blood fills up a few tubes. Within minutes, I'm back down the hall, out of the unit, through the sally port, onto the elevator, and down to the lab on the fourth floor. I know the Bangladeshi clerk at the window; he lets me take the blood directly back to the lab technicians instead of having to wait for him to do it. He can tell I am stressed out—I have beads of sweat on my forehead, my hands are a little shaky, and I'm talking faster than usual.

"Take a break, my dear," he calls out as I race back to the elevators. On the ride to the nineteenth floor in the empty elevator, I hold back the tears of exhaustion that are fighting to get out and take a few moments to breathe. Memories of my night with Rita, a patient from my internship year, flood my brain.

At the time I was covering the night shift for two weeks at Tisch Hospital, the NYU flagship medical facility one block north of Bellevue.

My partner for the shift was Colleen, a family-medicine intern. We mostly followed up lab values that were drawn during the day, checked on fever curves, and were generally available in case of an emergency. Rita's name was the last on the sign-out sheet that I received from the day team. The notation next to her name read, in all caps: "IF SHE HAS CHEST PAIN, GET AN ABG."

I didn't take much notice, spending the first few hours checking on patients, and when an elderly man on the tenth floor spiked a temperature, I headed off to culture his blood and get a urine sample. My pager went off as I was tying the tourniquet around his arm. Seventeenth-floor nursing station. I finished drawing the blood and stuck the samples in my coat pocket to drop off at the lab.

"Rita has chest pain," said Shelly, the pert and orderly blonde nurse on the seventeenth floor who was two years out of nursing school.

"OK," I replied, fumbling through my six-page sign-out to find out Rita's name. Who was she, again? Oh yeah, the ABG lady. ABG stood for arterial blood gas, a kind of blood draw that requires sticking a needle into an artery rather than a vein. I read the small-print details on the sign-out and saw that Rita had a history of several heart attacks as well as diabetes. She was in the hospital for a cardiac workup after coming to the ER multiple times in the previous week for chest pain of unknown etiology. Under the differential, someone had written "Anxiety?"

"Are her vital signs all right?" I asked.

"She's breathing fast and her blood pressure is up."

"On my way," I said, and hung up.

When I arrived, Rita looked like she was in pain. She was grabbing at her chest and taking short breaths, but her cardiac monitor wasn't showing much distress.

"Hi, Rita," I said. "I'm Dr. Ford. What's going on?" Rita was obese and looked much older than her thirty-five years.

"I . . . can't breathe . . ." she puffed. "The pain . . ."

"OK, OK, let me see here. Have you had the pain before?"

She nodded. I asked a few more questions, then proceeded to follow the directions in my sign-out.

"I'm going to check your blood oxygen levels to see whether we can figure this out. It's just a quick needle stick." Rita didn't know that I'd never done it before. Shelly, the nurse, clearly understood. She was used to having interns train on her units. She pulled me aside and gave me a quick and discreet tutorial, reminding me several times that if I stuck just a millimeter off the tiny radial artery in the wrist, I could hit the ulnar nerve and damage Rita's hand.

Back at Rita's bedside, I was all confidence and swagger.

"OK, here we go," I assured us both. I took a breath, steadied her arm on the bed, found the radial pulse at her wrist, and quickly plunged in the butterfly needle. Bright red blood filled the tube. I pulled out the needle, pressed some gauze on the tiny puncture wound, and exhaled. Success!

The tube went immediately into a cup of ice, and I headed down to the lab, tossing a quick thank-you to Rita over my shoulder. I was so excited about my first ABG that I thought little about Rita and her pain. I left her in her room, wheezing and gasping, as Shelly brought in some nitroglycerin to put under her tongue.

The lab processed the ABG quickly. Within minutes, I knew that Rita was just hyperventilating.

I headed back to her room and assured her that her heart looked fine. She was calm by then, but still looked upset.

"How do you know? The pain was so bad and it was here, on my left side," she motioned. "Shouldn't I get an EKG or something?"

"The cardiac monitor is looking good," I pointed out. "Try to get some rest. Let the nurse know if it happens again."

Around midnight, in the midst of checking the ventilator settings on a woman with emphysema, my beeper went off again, again from Shelly on the seventeenth floor, and again for Rita's chest pain. When I got to her, she looked exactly the same as she had before.

"It's happening again!" she shouted as I entered the room. "It's a heart attack! Do something!"

"Hold on, Rita; let me have a look. This is the same as last time?"

She nodded, clutching her chest.

"I have to take another blood gas," I sighed. "Sorry." I looked at the sign-out again to make sure I was actually supposed to draw another ABG.

The second needle stick went as smoothly as the first, and the results were the same.

"Nothing to worry about, Rita," I said as I arrived back in her room fifteen minutes later. "All looks good. Why don't you get some sleep?"

She didn't look reassured, but I didn't stick around to offer further comfort, either. I was done with my rounds for the night and desperately wanted to stretch out on the couch in the call room. Even a few minutes of sleep would help. I couldn't rest well during the days after my overnight shifts, so I tried to nap as much as possible at the hospital. I could usually get in a good hour or two of sleep each night.

Colleen was already asleep on one of the couches. I made myself a bed out of the linens piled in the corner and used my white coat as a blanket. I was afraid I'd sleep through my pager, so I clipped it onto my necklace, as close as possible to my ear. Within minutes, it went off.

I sat grumpily at the computer in the call room and typed in a few sleep-medication orders. More pages came in for various middle-of-the-night issues—one a call for Tylenol, a medication renewal that had been forgotten on the day shift. Every time I sat down at a computer to type orders, I began to doze off.

Around 4:00 a.m., my beeper went off again. Seventeenth floor. I called the nursing station.

"What?" I snapped when Shelly picked up the phone.

"You have to come up and draw another ABG on Rita," she said.

"Seriously?" I asked. "Have you tried just telling her to go to sleep?"

"No, I haven't, Dr. Ford," snipped Shelly. "Get up here."

"OK, OK, I'm coming." I threw some water on my face and stuffed a pack of M&M's in my pocket.

Rita was waiting for me.

"Hi, Dr. Ford, I was hoping you would come."

"I'm here," I said sharply. "Is anything different than the last couple of times I've been in here?"

"It's still so bad," she puffed. She looked desperate and pathetic, but I was not sympathetic.

"But is it different?" I pressed.

She conceded that it was not.

"OK, let's see your arm."

She held out her arm. She still had the gauze on her wrist from the last stick a few hours before. I pulled it off and was pleased that the puncture marks were barely visible—a sign of good technique.

This time, however, I missed the artery and stuck a vein instead. The deoxygenated blood that slowly filled the syringe was more deep purple than the bright red I wanted to see.

"Oh, crap," I muttered.

"What?" asked Rita nervously.

"Just missed the artery. Nothing to worry about. I'll try again and it should be fine."

She was surprisingly patient while I found another butterfly needle and pulled a spare tube from my pocket. The second attempt was successful but painful. Rita winced.

"Sorry," I said, although I was a little bit pleased that I had hurt her. "I have to get this to the lab, and you really need to get some sleep. Have you rested at all tonight?"

"I'm too afraid the pain will come back," she replied.

"Well, the good news is that so far, none of your test results show anything. Nothing to be afraid of."

"I'll try to get some sleep," she said quietly. She could tell that I was in no mood for conversation, and that I wanted more than anything to get out of her room.

"Great, thanks." Off I went to the lab, eager to catch some sleep before the day team interns began arriving in a few hours.

When the pager went off again, it wasn't about Rita, but a very simple request for Benadryl. That was all I could take. Tears of frustration started welling up and were in full force by the time I hung up the phone. I managed to write the order and then headed to the bathroom down the hallway. I locked the door and slumped in the corner.

"Dr. Ford, please come to the nursing station. Dr. Ford, you are needed at the seventeenth-floor nursing station." I heard Shelly on the overhead speaker but didn't move. Was she trying to get back at me for having been so rude earlier on the phone? I glanced at my pager and saw that I had missed a few pages in the last fifteen minutes, all from Shelly.

"Jesus," I thought to myself. "I can't do this anymore."

Yet, somehow, I stood up, wiped my nose with a bunch of toilet paper, and opened the door. Colleen was waiting outside with a look of pity.

"Can I help?" she asked.

"No, thanks," I quickly replied and scurried off, ashamed that she had seen me like that.

I couldn't even speak to Rita when I got to her room. I didn't ask about her symptoms; I just looked at the cardiac monitor—the same— and listened to her hyperventilate—the same. I was as out of control as Rita; I wanted to shake her and scream at her to get it together for both of us.

I motioned for her arm, and she silently laid it by her side. I put on my gloves, attached the needle to the tube, and missed her radial artery.

"Ow," she yelled. That was all I needed to head back over the edge.

"I'm sorry," I blubbered. "I am just so tired. Why do you have to keep calling me?" Tears clouded my vision and spattered onto her wrist. "I'll try it on the other side."

If I had been Rita, I would have pulled my wrist away and insisted that a more competent intern take over.

"Don't worry, Dr. Ford; you'll get it," Rita urged. "Just focus; you've done it before."

I listened to the calm and focused voice coming from the bed and couldn't believe it was Rita.

"Are you sure you want me doing this?" I sputtered, wiping my snotty nose on my scrub top.

"Definitely. You've been with me all night. I'd like to help you in return."

I took my time on her other wrist and marshaled every ounce of energy I had to keep my hands steady. She encouraged me the whole way, as focused on my success as I was. When the tube was filled and the tiny puncture site was covered in gauze, I looked up to find Rita breathing comfortably and sound asleep.

Now, almost three years later, the ding of the elevator reminds me that I'm back on the nineteenth floor.

"On the gate," I yell as soon as I get to the sally port. The control room officer responds more promptly this time.

"Hey, Dr. Ford," I hear from the other side of the gate. Officer Maddox is out of the intake area and heading toward me.

"You got to see Reynaldo," he says. "I don't think he can wait. And another one won't stop yelling."

"OK, but I've got a guy who had a fake seizure and won't get off the floor and another who just had a real seizure. Can I come in five minutes?"

"Don't think so," he says with a look of concern on his face. Officer Maddox has been in the DOC for close to twenty years, and working the intake pens for the past five. He's watched patients come off the midnight bus with broken jaws, bloody gashes—even a heart attack in progress. He knows when something bad is about to happen.

I follow him through a heavy unmarked door and into the holding area. Opposite a long stainless steel desk are three large intake pens. Each one has benches lining the walls and a molded toilet with parts that cannot be dismantled, partially obscured, with a waist-high privacy screen. The first two pens are quiet and dark. Reynaldo is in the last one, starting to bump his head against the wall. It is a gentle motion now, as though he's trying to massage his head against the concrete, but soon it's going to escalate. This is Reynaldo's warm-up for the violent skull crashing that—I learn when I read his chart—has landed him in the ICU on numerous occasions. He bangs his head against the wall because he has an IQ of 58 and doesn't know a better way to calm himself.

"Hey, hey, Reynaldo, come over here," I whisper through the bars. He doesn't respond. He is lost in his self-destructive soothing. I don't understand why someone like Reynaldo is even in jail—he functions at the level of a six-year old. He was picked up for smoking marijuana. He has been in and out of jail for two years, always arrested for misdemeanors, accumulating layers of scar tissue around his already sensitive brain every time he comes in. He doesn't know what he's done wrong; he just knows that he doesn't like it here. Banging his head helps, I suppose.

"Reynaldo, Reynaldo!" I say again, louder, pressing my face against the bars of the pen, hoping to break him out of his reverie. He stops momentarily and looks at me with wide brown eyes, then returns to knocking his head. I had hoped that I wouldn't have to admit him—an admission to the hospital takes a few hours, and I can usually get a patient back on the bus to Rikers Island in about twenty minutes—but it's not looking good.

"Get me the doctor!" I hear from around the corner in the hallway. There are three individual holding pens out there. The psychiatric patients usually get put out there because they get so agitated. Reynaldo is an exception because Officer Maddox knows how vulnerable he is.

The screaming in the hallway continues. "Get your fucking hands off me and get me the doctor! Now!"

I take my eyes off Reynaldo for a second and look around for Officer Maddox. He's heading toward the hallway, so I follow him out. I have no idea who the biggest emergency is—Bill on the floor on 19 West after his seizure, Reynaldo hitting his head on the concrete wall, or whoever this guy is in the hallway.

As soon as the screaming man sees me, he knows I'm the doctor. I'm the only one without a uniform, and the only woman. He's got two enormous men from the Department of Correction's ESU (Emergency Services Unit) team holding each of his arms, trying to get him back into his pen. ESU accompanies only the really dangerous patients.

"Hey, hey, Doc! Come over here! Do you see what they're doing? They can't do this to me! You got to tell them to stop!"

I look blankly at the scene. The patient's orange jumpsuit is sliding off one shoulder as he wrestles with the ESU; he looks tiny compared to the giants on either side of him. His long, curly black hair is tied back in a ponytail. It looks like there are some fresh cuts on his arms.

"I think you have to get back in the pen," I say meekly, trying not to piss anyone off, including the ESU. "I'm in the middle of talking to another patient; I'll be back as soon as I can."

"No, now!" he screams, just as I hear Reynaldo smash his head again.

I leave this mystery patient to fend for himself while I return to whispering to Reynaldo in an effort to get him to stop. This time, instead of head-banging, he starts rocking to the sound of my voice. I keep saying his name over and over while I look through the referral records from Rikers Island.

Reynaldo's been banging his head there, too. The overnight doc provided more details. "Other inmates taunting patient, telling him to bang his head, then laughing and encouraging him. Inmate needs evaluation for his own safety." I know that whoever becomes Reynaldo's doctor on Monday will be annoyed that I admitted him. He's intellectually disabled and doesn't have an illness that medication in the hospital will fix. He'll be one of those patients that the staff will have to watch all the time like a child. But I can't send him back to the jail. I just can't. He's sitting down on the bench now, rocking.

"We're going to admit him," I tell Officer Maddox. "I'll do the paperwork in a bit. I'm heading back to 19 West now to take care of the seizure. I'll get the nurses to bring Reynaldo over quickly so that we can get him calmed down. Will you keep an eye on him? If he starts banging his head again, page me."

"You got it. What about the screamer out there?" he says as he motions to the hallway.

"I guess he'll keep screaming. I promise I'll get back as soon as possible."

Back on 19 West, Pedro has gotten tired of the cold tile floor and returned to his bed. The hallways are empty. One of the aides is watching Bill in his room. He seems to have regained consciousness and is resting.

"Hey, Anne, how's it going?" I ask as I enter the nursing station. She doesn't look great. Anne is in her mid-fifties, with graying curly hair that was probably luxurious when she was younger. She carries around a fanny pack full of tissues and bottles of medication prescribed for her by the many doctors she visits—I don't know what for.

"How do you think?" she replies sarcastically, although it doesn't feel mean.

"Yeah, I hear you," I say. "Let me just check Bill's labs—they should be back by now."

"Help! Help!" I hear from down the hallway. "He's having another seizure!"

My heart is already pounding out of fear for Reynaldo; now it starts thumping even louder. I find Bill on the floor of his room, shaking with a violent rhythm, his eyes rolled back in his head.

"Call a code!" I yell to Anne. "And get that Ativan!"

Within minutes, the airway team and the medical consult arrive to help stabilize Bill. Even after the shot of Ativan, he's still seizing. Someone inserts an IV into his arm—a procedure not usually allowed on the forensic psychiatry service because the tubing can serve as a noose—and he starts to get mainline sedatives. The medical consult arranges for Bill's immediate transfer out of the unit and into the ICU. I watch as he gets loaded onto a gurney, his hands cuffed to the railing. It reminds me of the stories I have heard of pregnant inmates being shackled during labor.

I wipe my sweaty forehead and sigh in relief. Bill is one less patient for me to worry about. Reynaldo is a different story, but he's unlikely to end up in the ICU. He needs a one-to-one watch, someone to stay on him like a shadow, and a good night's sleep. Whoever comes on during the day can figure out a more solid plan. Only five more hours before my shift is over at 9:00 a.m. I am starting to feel nauseated with fatigue.

There is still the problem of the screaming patient in the intake area. Officer Maddox tells me that he has been yelling on and off ever since I left.

"Doc! Why has it taken you so long?" the patient greets me when I return. "I can't take this much longer." He shows me the dried blood on his arms.

"What's your name?" I ask, just wanting to get this encounter over with.

"Peter."

"How old are you?"

"Twenty-eight."

"Why'd they bring you to the hospital?"

He starts from the beginning, and I try to keep the details straight. There was a fight with another inmate about respect; when officers came to intervene, Peter spit in their faces. The team of officers came down hard on him. He ended up in "the box"—punitive segregation, or solitary confinement—and has been there for more than six months.

He describes being locked in a 7 x 12 ft. cell with a thin mattress on a bed frame, a small sink and toilet in one corner, a louvered window covered in fine mesh, and a heavy, remote-controlled steel door with a slot for meal deliveries three times a day. Although he was entitled to an hour out of his cell each day, the officers rarely had the handcuffs and shackles required to escort him out, so he didn't go. Instead, Peter says, he screamed through the slot, drew pictures on his walls with leftover sauce from his food tray, and mutilated his body in whatever way he could tolerate so that he could be taken out of his cell to the medical clinic.

"That sounds pretty awful," I concede, "but why did someone send you to the psychiatric hospital?"

He shows me his arms. "I can't take it anymore," he says softly. "You got to help me. I can't stay in the box."

I ask him a few more questions, and he answers the right way to get himself an admission.

"Do you want to kill yourself now?"

"Yes."

"Do you have a plan?"

"Sure do," he says. "You ever seen the place over there?" referring to Rikers Island. I shake my head no.

"The buildings are all falling apart. AMKC, man," he says—short for the Anna M. Kross Center, named after the DOC commissioner from 1954 to 1966—"that place is a hole." It is the largest and most decrepit of the jails on the Island.

"There's leaks dripping everywhere in that place," Peter continues, "and tiles peeling off the floor. It ain't hard to get something sharp. Hey, half the jail wants me to kill myself anyway."

The ESU officers sitting along the hallway shake their heads in frustration. One of them covers his mouth and coughs, "Bullshit."

I don't have the energy to explore whether Peter's accounting is accurate. I don't really care. He's lucky tonight.

"I'm going to admit you, Peter," I say, stifling a yawn. "But listen, it's gonna take a few hours to get all the paperwork done. Will you please just rest for a while and try to be quiet?"

"Doc, you won't regret this," he says. "I owe you."

"You don't owe me anything," I sigh. "Just please try to behave on the unit. They'll discharge you real fast if you get in a fight."

He nods and promises something that he probably cannot deliver.

By the time I've documented my night in the notes and orders in the charts for Pedro, Bill, Reynaldo, and Peter, the sun is up and shining through the wire mesh covering the windows. I trudge down to the CPEP to drop off the pager so the next shift's moonlighter can pick it up. I'm also eager to see Marc, the former chief resident from 19 North, before he signs out in the CPEP. Marc is now an attending there and works the Friday overnight shift. He's my backup, in case I get into trouble on the floors upstairs. He is also, by now, my boyfriend.

On the way in, I pass two NYPD cops and two EMTs, one of whom is pushing a rickety wooden wheelchair that carries a very angry Black man who's strapped in with a cloth tie around his chest. I can't make out what he's yelling about. His hands are cuffed behind his back and wedged between the wooden slats of the back of the chair. His ankles are shackled to the footrests. He's probably going to be the next admission to 19 West.

I don't find Marc, so I stumble the four blocks home and sink into my couch; I'm asleep within seconds. When I wake up hours later in the middle of a chilly Saturday afternoon, I know that I'm done with this moonlighting job. I can't take another night like last night. There's too much pain up there, I think, too much panic. It's going to mess with my head if I don't stop.

4

NEVER WHAT YOU EXPECT

Another year passes, and I'm finishing up my residency and thinking about my career. I have forgotten the panic and pain on the nineteenth floor. I remember only the pace, the excitement, the powerful feeling of being a front-line doctor trying to help her patients. The further away I get from the nineteenth floor, the more romantic my memories become. I remember Officer Maddox, screaming Peter, frazzled Anne, and seizing Bill fondly, as though they're friends. I want to get back there.

On July 1, 2004, I start a fellowship in forensic psychiatry. In this yearlong postresidency training program, I learn about things like testifying in court, insanity evaluations, sex offenders, involuntary hospitalization, and even negotiation tactics from *The Art of War*. My first clinical rotation lands me right back on 19 West.

As a fellow, I am now almost an attending. I need to get all of my patient notes cosigned by an attending, but I can do therapy, write medication orders, and make clinical decisions basically on my own. It helps that I know a lot of the nursing staff already from those Friday overnights I used to do. My first day of fellowship, listening at rounds about the patients on the unit, I learn that Peter is back.

He's actually been back here a few times in the fourteen months since I saw him last. He's still in jail on the same charge and still struggling to hold it together. He's also still in punitive segregation but is now on a unit called MHAUII (Mental Health Assessment Unit for Infracted Inmates), pronounced like the island in Hawaii. MHAUII was designed as a more treatment-oriented form of segregation with the opportunity to earn extra hours out of one's cell for good behavior. The idea was solid—positive reinforcement—but the practice was not. Within several years of opening, MHAUII was indistinguishable from regular solitary confinement.

This time, Peter had been admitted from Rikers Island for swallowing a "soap ball," a tidy packet given to inmates to clean their cells that contains highly concentrated detergent and bleach. He was probably trying to get out of MHAUII. Splashing bodily fluids through the food slot, swallowing foreign objects, and self-mutilation are common in there.

Peter's been at Bellevue for a few days, and today he's headed back to the Island, as soon as his doctor can get him out. Yesterday, he pushed past several nurses and, half-naked, chased another patient down the hallway and threatened to cut out his tongue. I am not going to see Peter today, but I am sure that I will see him again sometime soon.

One of my assignments as a fellow is to lead a community meeting in the morning with as many of the patients and staff as possible. We try to arrange it right after breakfast, when everyone is already seated around the six bolted-down picnic tables in the dining room.

I go to the front of the room next to the TV, also bolted to the ground in its custom-built, tamper-resistant case.

"Good morning, gentlemen. Today is Wednesday, July 27, and this is our community meeting. Can someone tell me the rules of the meeting?"

A few hands immediately go up. These mostly belong to patients who have been here for a month or more.

"Yes, sir?" I point to one.

"Keep it to community issues!"

"Great, thanks. Yes, if you have issues that relate just to you, like your treatment or your legal case, please save that for your individual sessions."

"No cross-talk!" I hear from the back of the room.

"Right," I confirm; each inmate gets time to talk without interruption. "And you are reminding me of another rule. Please raise your hand and wait to be called on if you would like to say something. Any more rules?"

From the back of the room again, "If you have to go to the bathroom, you can't come back."

"Well, I guess that's basically correct. It's not a very long meeting, so we ask that if you have to get up to leave for any reason—even if that's going to the bathroom—you don't return. Helps limit the disruptions."

I look around to see whether anyone wants to add any more rules, and then I open the floor to issues. Mostly I hear about the dirty showers, the flimsy pajamas, and frustration with the DOC. I try to nudge these meetings in the direction of therapy—"What is it like to be in a hospital that is also a jail?" Instead I usually get a response about the lack of soap or the need for a new Ping-Pong table. Not a lot of sharing of feelings.

Kareem, one of the patients, raises his hand and stands up tall, unfurling his long legs out from under the picnic table. His voice is deep and thundering, and he talks about the three volumes of a book he is writing, something about a phoenix and God—"the next Bible," he says.

I try to interrupt him, but he keeps going.

"I'm not done yet. Don't shut me up."

One of the officers standing outside of the dining room starts to walk in when he hears Kareem raise his voice.

"Hey, hey, I ain't gonna hurt her, man!" he yells. "That ain't my style. Stop freaking out. Just let me finish my thought."

I look around the room as if the patients are going to give me some advice about how to handle this situation. Some of them are asleep and a few are talking to themselves, but everyone else has full attention on Kareem and the officer, waiting to see if there is going to be a fight.

"OK, Kareem, go ahead." I take a few steps back, as if to offer him the floor. "But try to keep it brief." I look over at the officer, who is now leaning against the wall with his hands folded across his chest. He's a good fifteen inches shorter than Kareem but looks like he lifts weights.

Several minutes go by, and Kareem is still expounding. He doesn't seem to be losing any steam.

"Hey, man, can you sit down?" asks one of the patients who's been on the unit for a while. "We're supposed to talk about community issues, not your book."

"It's a community issue, man," Kareem responds. "You guys are all going to read it someday."

I let out a chuckle and the room goes silent as everyone looks at the new doctor who's laughing at Kareem.

"I hope we all get to read it someday," I recover, looking Kareem right in the eye. "But we'll never do that if we don't finish up this community meeting and let everyone talk."

"Guess you're right," Kareem concedes. He sits down, tucking his legs back under the table.

After the meeting, I find Kareem in his room organizing the hundreds of sheets of paper that he assures me will eventually turn into his book. He grabs a seemingly random handful, puts them in order, and shoves them in my direction.

"Hey, Doc, you've got to read this. This is the first thirty-seven pages. Tell me it isn't a bestseller."

The pages are stained with something unrecognizable, and some of them are ripped and falling apart.

"That's OK, Kareem," I protest, uninterested in touching those pages with my bare hands. "Maybe later you can read me some?"

"No, no, you've got to read it. In your office. Here, take it." The pages are now only a few inches from my chest, and I start to wonder whether Kareem is going to hit me with them. I reach out my hand and grab the wrinkled stack.

"OK, OK, I'll read these," I say. "But if I do, you and I have to talk about medication." Kareem was good at talking his way out of taking medication, but he really needed it to control his bipolar disorder.

"The deal maker!" he cries. "Nothing gets past you, huh?"

I shrug. "Deal?"

"You got me, Doc. Deal. But you have to give me a book report before we talk about Depakote." Smiling, we shake on it.

Back in my office, I photocopy the pages and put the originals in a folder to go back to Kareem. Then I scrub my hands twice with disinfectant soap before sitting down to read the clean pages. They're filled with writing about the devil, God, and the world according to Kareem. When I return to the unit, I stumble through an attempt to summarize for him what I have just read. He can tell that I'm struggling.

"That's OK, Doc. I can tell you don't get it. You aren't one of the chosen ones, like me. There aren't many of us out there. But I can see that you read it. So what do you want to ask me about meds?"

At the end of the day, I walk a few blocks west to a private office I share with another young psychiatrist, Ella. She's a close friend from residency who is training to be a psychoanalyst. We each have a handful of patients who come to see us every week. I like the feeling of running my own business, scheduling my own time, and working in an office that has nice armchairs and its own fax machine. I think I'm supposed to enjoy this work more than what I do in the grimy holding pens at Bellevue—my supervisors and colleagues all rave about the autonomy and the money—but I find myself uncomfortable during these private office sessions, as if my patients are strangers and each time I see them it is for the first time.

I tell no one about this discomfort. I am too ashamed to admit that I am more attached to patients like Kareem and Peter. My aunt says the same thing I hear from most of my colleagues and friends: "I'll never understand why you like to work with those prisoners." I can't articulate it to her—or, at this point, even to myself—but there is an unmistakable sense of purpose and connection with my Bellevue patients, a lack of pretense. They know that I can't get them out of jail or give them a job or a home. I can give them my time, though, and that seems to be all they expect. No miracles here. The conversations I have with them are some of the most real and honest in my life.

5

THE TENDER AND THE TROUBLED

Nineteen North, the unit I remember most for my battle with Dr. Miller over Mary and my flirtations with Marc, now a psychoanalyst in private practice, my husband as of a year ago, and the father of our four-month-old son—underwent a multimillion-dollar maximum security transformation. It became part of the Bellevue Hospital Prison Ward in 2004, adding an additional twenty-eight psychiatric beds to the forty beds already on 19 West. The makeover included bars on the windows, breaker gates in the hallway to shut off sections in case of a riot, shatterproof glass for the nursing station, and officers guarding the doors and posted in the unit.

Gate 7 is now the first port of entry. It's a confusing entrance. When I started working on 19 North as the unit chief, or head psychiatrist, only a few months after my fellowship ended, I made the rookie mistake of pressing a large red button on the wall labeled "Push to Open." It sounded a loud and unpleasant buzz about twenty-five feet away in a small foyer where Officer Dennis, the "A" post officer, sat. She looked at me through her Plexiglas panel and went back to writing in her logbook. I buzzed again, not sure of what was supposed to happen. This time she completely ignored me. I stood there, helpless and bewildered, until another officer walked by. He radioed the control room over by 19

West, and within seconds, the gate started to open. When I finally made it to Officer Dennis in the foyer, she scolded me for pushing the button.

"But it says . . ."

"You believe everything you read?" she interrupted.

My first lesson as unit chief: never touch the red button.

This morning, I make it into the unit without any problem. Officer Dennis and I have made nice, and she's apparently forgiven my red-button error. I head into the conference room, a small classroom-size space, mostly consumed by a large table in the middle that's surrounded by straight-backed chairs. A giant whiteboard with the remnants of notes from a psychology lecture about personality styles hangs on one wall; stacked boxes of photocopied blank documents—patient consent forms, admission forms, nursing assessments—are piled against the other wall. A computer sits broken and silent in one corner, kept company only by a rumpled Fritos wrapper and a Coke can, left here overnight by whichever officer took a break—and a nap—in the room.

As usual, the team is already assembled by the time I come rushing in after dropping my son at daycare at 8:00 a.m., having frantically hailed a cab to get me down the east side of Manhattan to the hospital.

The team is loudly chattering and laughing around the table when I walk into the conference room. The volume quickly drops, papers start to be organized, and a few people sit up a little straighter when they see me. Ever since my son was born, my tolerance for work chitchat and inefficiency has decreased considerably. I am on the clock now, with only eight hours and twenty-five minutes before I have to be back out on First Avenue, hailing a cab to get me back uptown to daycare. I sometimes miss my old self in these moments, remembering all the joking and laughter I used to share during rounds as a resident, planning for drinks after work or gossiping about boyfriends and cute attendings. The team now respects my passion for the work, but I'm pretty sure they wish I were a little more laid-back about it.

I sit down at the head of the conference table with Marie, the charge nurse for the day, to my left. Marie is a sturdy and outspoken Haitian nurse who has been at Bellevue for decades. Her job at rounds is to report on what has happened overnight, to tell us who refused to take his medication, who got into an argument with the staff, who was up all night. Next to Marie sits Luke, the other psychiatrist who works on 19 North. He is a good balance for my opinionated intensity. Luke is soft-spoken and keeps his comments to himself. He never complains about too much work, never appears flustered or tired.

To Luke's left around the table sit—in positions that never seem to change—a sixty-five-year-old case worker named John, several psychology students, one of two psychologists, a medical student, an art therapist, and, to my immediate right, another psychologist. John has worked at Bellevue for forty years and has created a niche for himself as the guy who knows legal details. Since the patients all want to know their next court date or how to reach their attorney, I covet John's clipboard, crowded with lists of New York penal codes, Legal Aid attorney phone numbers, and patient rap sheets. I also have a soft spot for John. He has an awkward, mumbling style about him, but he works hard and cares deeply.

"Good morning, everyone," I say, reaching for the photocopied list of patients on the unit and trying to sound casual and fun, since I had just killed the laughter with my entrance.

"Good morning," is the subdued response I get in return.

"Sorry to be late," I continue. "Thanks for waiting. Marie, should we get started?"

"Sure, whatever you like," replies Marie. Her tone is snippy and curt, but I've come to learn that everything she says has this edge.

She goes through the patients, describing some as "OK, no problems," and others as "a mess." We spend more time as a team discussing the messes, including Jamel, one of my patients, who was admitted only a few days before. Marie tells me that he is "stable" but that he is waiting for me with bloody arms in the treatment room on the unit.

"Bloody arms?" I ask, alarmed.

Marie assures me that he can wait until rounds are over, and begins to introduce the new patients who have been admitted since yesterday. It's one of my jobs to assign them to either Luke or myself, and to our respective clinical teams. Today is easy—two new patients, one per team. I hurry us through the rest of rounds, talking about discharges, plans for the new admissions, group therapy happening that day, and patients around whom the students should be particularly cautious.

"Thanks, everyone," I say. "I think that's it for now. I'm going to head in and see Jamel." As I leave the room, I see Luke rally his team around the corner of the table and start to figure out plans for the day.

After a quick hello at the nursing station, I head into the treatment room, sparkly evidence of the recent 19 North renovation. It's spacious and clean, with shiny stainless steel supply cabinets, a full range of office medical equipment that includes a new EKG machine and examining table, and a portable oxygen supply. Jamel and his bloody arms are indeed waiting for me. A DOC officer I've never met before is standing at the open doorway and steps aside to let me through.

I stare at Jamel's arms and try to understand the mess of scratches and tears on his skin. They are in various states of healing, some with fresh, red blood oozing onto his flimsy, hospital-issue pajamas, and others covered by thick keloid knots a few shades lighter than his blue-black skin. One of the wounds is starting to look a little red, and when I put my gloved hand on his skin, it feels warm and throbbing. Jamel doesn't seem to notice. He is listening to something that I can't hear.

I look up and see Eric through the small, square window in the mostly closed treatment room door. I feel safe. Eric is one of the nursing techs assigned to manage the floor and talk to patients when they are getting agitated—"verbal de-escalation," as it's called. Eric and I have a kind of soul connection from my early days of residency, when he helped teach me how to talk to patients in the CPEP. He is a hulk of a man who treats the patients gently, as though they were his own children. I glance at him again through the shatterproof glass, then turn back to Jamel and his bloody arms. My fleeting feeling of safety is gone.

"What's he doing out there?" Jamel snarls from the examination table, glaring past me at Eric.

"I don't want no black person staring at me; he ain't got no right to do that." His voice gets louder. "Did you tell him to be out there? You scared of me, Doc? Huh, you scared?" He is almost yelling. If Jamel's voice goes a decibel louder, Eric is going to come storming in and insist that the examination is over. I put my arm up to stop Eric and give him a thumbs up. Please don't come in, I think. I need Jamel to trust me. So despite my pounding heart and an urge to run, I do what I think is best. I tell Jamel the truth.

"Yeah, Jamel," I whisper, "I'm scared." My voice gradually comes back to me, and I continue. "I wasn't scared before, when I was just looking at your arms for an infection, but now I am. I don't want to be, but I can't help it. It's scary to have you scream in my face." I take a few steps back as I speak, and bump into the blood pressure cuff on the wall. I let out a yelp as the cuff tumbles off its hook and lands on my shoulder. Jamel explodes in a deep, throaty laugh as I fumble around trying to hide my embarrassment.

"You ain't got to worry, Doc," he chuckles. "Just keep that gorilla out of the room and we'll be fine."

"No one's coming in here unless they need to," I say softly. "Now let's have a look at your arms again." He fidgets a little before resting his forearms in my outstretched hands. "How did all of this happen?"

"I dunno," Jamel answers. "I try to tell them to stop, but they don't listen to me. It's like every morning I've got this black stuff all over me again. Like dirt or somethin'. Shower doesn't get it off no matter how hard I scrub."

I have no idea what he is talking about.

"Can you show me the stuff? Do you have any of it anywhere now?" Jamel looks at me with impatience.

"Doc, are you blind? It's all over me. Look."

He starts peeling at the tender skin over his wrist, digging his long thumbnail next to a bumpy vein and flicking off whatever pieces of flesh he can remove.

"Wait, wait," I say. "Don't do that, please." I get a few Band-Aids out of the supply cabinet and smooth them over his wrist. I pretend that I understand what he is telling me, and hope that the more he talks, the clearer it will become.

"How long has this been happening to you?" I prompt.

"Maybe a few years," he says. He is twenty-four years old now; a few years before would be perfect timing for the onset of schizophrenia.

"How did it start?"

"Kind of slow, at first. I thought it was a skin condition, like what's that thing that Michael Jackson has? When his skin started turning white? Well, like, I thought I had that in reverse."

I nod, encouraging him to keep talking. "Did you go see any doctors for it?" I ask, casually heading over to the cabinet to get supplies to draw his blood. I am pretty sure he is harboring an infection in a few of the cuts on his arm.

"Yeah. They just sent me to see the psych. Waste of time. One of the doctors in the ER was working for them. He tried to give me the needle and put me to sleep. He probably thought I didn't notice, but I had him pegged from the moment I walked in. Don't worry—I got him."

"Is that why you got arrested?" I ask. I know from his admission paperwork that he has been arrested on a serious assault charge—the doctor he hit had to spend five hours in surgery.

"That ain't nothin'," he says. "I can get out of jail anytime I want. Sometimes I like it in here because I get a break from all the problems outside. It's also harder for them to find me in here."

"Them?" I ask.

Jamel glances at Eric again and then looks at the floor, silent.

"Jamel?" I prod, bending down so I can look up at his face.

He remains silent, but his fists start to ball up. I back away.

"Hey, no problem," I say, trying to sound relaxed. "Why don't we just get you cleaned up? We can talk later."

"It's not you, Doc," he says. "I just don't want you to get hurt. Maybe they'll come after you if I tell you too much. They watch me all the time."

"You can't tell me who?" I urge. I am pushing too hard and yet I am so curious that I can't keep my mouth shut.

He clenches his jaw and shakes his head.

"Wish I could tell you. Just please, will you help me get this stuff off?" He starts picking at his skin again.

"Your skin?" I ask, still confused. "Help you get your skin off?"

"I knew it," he suddenly fumes, jumping off the table and ripping the Band-Aids off his arm. "You don't believe me either! You think I'm crazy, just like the rest of them. I ain't standin' for that. I'm as white as you are, so don't think that you can pull this high-and-mighty bullshit on me just because you're a doctor. Get the hell out of my face!"

He only gets a few steps past me and toward the door before Eric is in the room.

"Hey, Jamel, it's cool, man," he purrs. "Ain't no problem here. Let's just get back to your room." He starts to put his hand on Jamel's shoulder.

"Get the fuck off me, man!" Jamel yells. "All y'all, just leave me alone."

He pushes past Eric, runs past the nursing station window, and heads across the hall into his bedroom. A couple of nurse's aides and a curious medical student in a short white coat follow him. Eric makes sure I am steady on my feet and then takes off as well. I stay behind in the treatment room to catch my breath. I could have been another casualty of Jamel's psychosis. Instead, I feel pride—I feel exhilaration. Jamel could easily have knocked me unconscious, but he chose to keep me safe.

At night, at home, a little bit of that exhilaration helps me get through what has become a baseline of exhaustion. I go to sleep every night with the shadow of my three-inch pager next to my bed. Last weekend, while pushing my son on a playground swing in Central Park, I was on the phone the whole time, talking down the covering doctor who had just witnessed two patients fight and sent one of them down to X-ray for a possible facial fracture.

Marc worries about me, I think, but he tries to keep it to himself. When I tell him about Jamel, after our son has eaten and is lying in my arms in a postprandial nap, Marc's brow crinkles in the way that lets me know he's anxious.

"You sure everything is OK?" he asks. "It hasn't been that long since you've been back at work from maternity leave."

"Yeah, everything's fine," I say, no hint left of the energy from the day. I wish I hadn't said anything about Jamel.

"It was a little scary, but I don't think he actually wanted to hurt me. Eric was there, just in case."

Marc knows Eric from his days in the CPEP, and I know that if I mention his name, Marc will feel more comfortable about the work I do. I don't want to feel the weight of his worry.

"I have to pump," I say, slowly shifting our son to the bassinet and hoping that he stays asleep for at least a half hour. Pumping breast milk for my son's bottles buys me some of the only solitude I can find each day and allows me to avoid, at least for now, Marc's crinkled brow.

6

MAMA GRIZZLY

Kevin is the new guy. He has the unfortunate luck of living in only one of two states in this country—the other being North Carolina—where anyone sixteen years of age or older is automatically charged as an adult. He is sixteen, but his small, scrawny body makes him look about twelve.

Kevin came in from the Adolescent Reception and Detention Center (ARDC, since renamed RNDC for former DOC chief Robert N. Davoren). It houses the adolescent boys, and, as I would learn years later from exposés like "The Lords of Rikers" (*New York* magazine, 2011) and "Before the Law" (*The New Yorker*, 2014), is perhaps the most lawless and dangerous jail on the Island. Christopher Robinson will be beaten to death there in 2008 and Kalief Browder will eventually kill himself after spending over a year in solitary confinement for a stolen backpack, for which he was never found guilty.

Kevin hasn't been in solitary confinement yet. The only thing on his mind today is the phone. The phone is always a problem for the jail patients at Bellevue. It is never fair and never easy. One of the floor officers is supposed to bring the phone and cord into the unit at 8:00 a.m. and make it available for patients until late in the evening. It's an old-model white Trimline with the numbers on the handset. There is no cradle, just a long cord attached to the end. The cord plugs into the one available wall jack so that it can be removed at the end of the day and won't be used as a weapon. Whenever the phone is in use, an officer is usually standing a few feet away, making sure that the caller isn't turning the cord into a noose. Each patient is supposed to get one six-minute personal call and one attorney phone call per day. Unlike at Rikers Island, where the phone automatically clicks off when time is up, at Bellevue, the officers are responsible for keeping time.

Manuel, another patient, usually gets a lot of time on the phone and likes to spend it whispering to his baby mama about what he wants to do to her body once he gets out. He is sweet to the female officers and submissive with the men; this seems to get him extra phone time. He was arrested on a drug charge while he was intoxicated and doesn't have much of a mental health history. I don't know how he got admitted, and I hope he won't be here long. But now that he is here and sober, he keeps threatening suicide so that we won't send him to Rikers Island.

Manuel is on the phone when I go to find Kevin in the rec room. My footsteps slap through the shiny new unit. Officer Brown, a ten-year veteran of the prison ward and a cool cat under pressure, greets me with a warm smile as I walk by. I have only been on the service for about six months, but not once have I heard Officer Brown raise his voice. The hallway is a natural amplifier, so it always sounds loud and chaotic. Officer Brown's soft voice is very comforting.

The rec room is a large open area that connects 19 West and 19 North. The room has a beautiful northward view up the East River, obstructed only by the fine mesh covering the windows. We sometimes have community meetings in here, but otherwise, it's a common area where patients can get away from the clinical space of the unit. The more functional patients are playing checkers or Ping-Pong; others are tucked in a corner talking or laughing to themselves, or watching the large TV.

I find Kevin staring out the window at the glistening United Nations building up the river. He has one big, expressive eye that opens wide with fear and scrunches when he tries to laugh; I can't see the other eye, because it is sealed shut with swollen and bruised skin.

"Oh, my goodness!" I exclaim. "What happened?"

He turns his face away and doesn't respond. I wait there, figuring that he will talk when he is ready. Out of the corner of my eye I see Emile, my patient with a movement disorder, flailing his arms in the middle of the room. I've been trying to move Emile onto the neurology service so they can figure out whether his motor tics are a result of a seizing brain or more of a psychosomatic response to the stresses of being in jail. He's a handful.

Eventually, Kevin turns to me and starts to giggle.

"You going to ask me anything else, Doc, or just stand there staring at me? Seems kinda weird."

I smile in relief.

"I have a million questions for you," I reply. "You want to talk someplace more private, or are you OK in here?"

"Here's good. I don't want to go back in there," he says, motioning back to the unit.

I nod and begin. "How about we start with why you ended up in the hospital."

"You tell me. I didn't ask to come in here. I was just mindin' my business when they threw me on the bus and sent me over. Seriously, I stick to myself over there," referring to ARDC.

"Were you seeing a doctor at Rikers?" I ask. "A psychiatrist, maybe?"

"Yeah, I went to the clinic sometimes," he slowly replies. "They just kept askin' me the same dumb questions. Shit like, was I thinking of killin' myself and how was I sleepin'. Waste of time. Like I'm gonna talk about any of that."

"When was the last time you went to that clinic?"

He shrugs his shoulders and looks down again.

"Hey, don't worry," I say. "You're here now; that's good. First up, though, we've got to talk about your eye. Does it hurt?"

He nods silently.

"When did it happen?"

"Don't matter," he mumbles. "It ain't nothin'."

"I don't know," I say. "I've seen a lot of black eyes. That one looks pretty bad."

By now I can spot an orbital fracture a mile away, the bruising and swelling masking the broken, fragile bones that protect the eyeball. A lot of my patients have these microfractures, either coming in with them following a "use of force" at Rikers Island or after a fight with another patient.

"I'm going to order an X-ray just to make sure nothing is broken. Maybe get you some pain medication. You OK with that?"

He stares at his hands and is quiet again. I don't know whether he has heard me or whether he is scared to talk about his eye in such a public setting. I repeat my question.

"Yeah, that's OK," he says softly. "But I want to talk to my mom. She don't know I'm in here, and I want to make sure she knows where I'm at. When can I call her? I don't want to talk to you no more."

His words sting a bit.

"How about we talk for a few more minutes, and then we get you signed up for the phone? DOC controls it, so just get your name on the list and they'll call you when it's your turn."

"Where is the list? Who do I ask?" he presses, clearly not interested in talking to me about anything else.

"I'll show you when we're done," I say, frustration leaking into my voice.

"Come on; can we be done?" he pleads.

"I still don't know much about you . . ."

"I know, I know," he interrupts, "but I got to call my mom. She's gonna worry."

"OK," I finally concede. I am not getting anything else out of him now. "We can finish this afternoon. Let's go get you a phone call."

We leave the dayroom, pass Manuel on the phone, and look for the officer in charge. My heart sinks. Officer Manor is a particular problem in our unit. Unlike the rest of the officers, she is just plain mean. She is a tall, beautiful black woman but calls any patient who comes too close to her a "crazy nigger." She acts as though the patients in the unit are part of a different species.

"Hi, Officer Manor," I cheerfully begin, approaching her perch on a cheap plastic chair next to the rec room.

"I'm busy; hold on," she replies in a gruff tone, taking what seems like a really long time to write something in her logbook. She eventually looks up.

"Yeah, what?" she snaps.

"This is Kevin," I say, pointing to him. "He's never been here before and would like to call his mom. Can you help get him on the phone list and explain how it works?"

"Who are you?" she asks, fixing Kevin with her eyes.

"I'm Kevin," he softly replies.

"Last name?" she barks.

He gives it and stands there, waiting for her to tell him what to do next. She writes his name in the book and turns away.

"What do I do now?" he asks.

"You wait till I call you and you keep your mouth shut."

I also keep my mouth shut and usher Kevin back to his room.

"They aren't all like that; I promise," I say. "Just try to be patient. You're sort of down the list, so it might be a while before your phone call. But you'll get it; I promise. Maybe check back with Officer Manor in an hour."

He nods and sits on his bed. Everything in Kevin's room, in all of the rooms, is as suicide- and weapon-proof as possible. The blue-green beds and cubbies, the only pieces of furniture, are made of thick plastic that can't be whittled into shanks. The beds are secured to the floor with tamper-proof screws, the kind that can't be loosened and swallowed. A thin, floppy mattress lies on top of each bed, covered with rubberized fabric stitched inside out so the threads can't easily be removed and the mattress fabric ripped into strips. There are no pillows allowed on the unit; the mattress is shaped so that there is slightly more filling at the head. Each patient gets one thin sheet and, in the winter, a scratchy gray blanket.

I leave Kevin looking at the floor and go to the nursing station to write some notes. The nursing station is a large room, more spacious and clean than the much older space on 19 West. The 19 North unit is a giant "L" of a hallway, with the entrance near the top of the L and the nursing station closer to the bend. The one nursing station door, along with the treatment room, is down a short corridor off the main hallway, protected from patient entry by a thin red line painted on the floor. The red lines are scattered throughout the unit, warning patients to stop and get permission before crossing over into areas close to the exit or within earshot of clinical spaces like interview or activity rooms. Patients may not always respect each other or the staff, but they pay attention to those lines.

The front wall of the nursing station has glass paneling with a direct view of the four "high observation" rooms, located to be always visible and under more intensive observation that the other rooms in the unit. Kevin is in one of these rooms because he is so young. Adolescents are prime targets in jail for all kinds of abuse, from stealing a PIN code used to pay for phone calls to rape. We can't change the law that allows sixteen-year-olds to be in jail—yet—but we can at least try to protect Kevin while he is here.

I rifle through Kevin's chart, looking for anything that will help me. I don't find much. A few sentences from the referring doctor saying that Kevin had stopped eating a few days before and wasn't leaving his cell. No mention of the black eye.

Luke, the other psychiatrist, is sitting in a rolling chair, renewing medication orders for one of his patients. Anne, the nurse who shared many Friday overnight shifts with me years before, is in the medication

room prepping the afternoon doses of Risperdal and Zoloft. She is muttering about the amount of work she has ahead of her. I go over to one of
the two computers bolted to the counter and look to see whether Kevin
had his blood drawn when he got admitted. All of the new patients to
the unit are supposed to get blood tests to check for things that can
cause psychiatric illnesses, including thyroid disease, low sodium, and
high glucose; urine tests to screen for drugs and make sure the kidneys
are working properly; and a chest X-ray to rule out tuberculosis. According to the computer, Kevin never had his blood work ordered. I'll
have to take care of that before the end of the day, I think, and reach
for another patient's chart.

Within a few minutes, I hear Officer Manor shouting.

"Stop coming up to me, you crazy kid! I said I'd call you when the
phone was ready. Get back in your room and stay away from me or I
won't give you your call. Just try me!"

I can see through the glass that Kevin is out of his room and looking confused. "But he's been on the phone forever," he says, pointing at
Manuel.

Officer Manor smirks at Kevin while Manuel gives him the finger.
Kevin skulks back to his bedroom.

After another five minutes, he is out again.

"I really need to call my mom," he pleads again.

"You ain't gettin' no phone call now," she shouts, crossing his name
off the logbook. "Get away from me!"

Kevin starts to get desperate.

"Please, please, I need to call her. She don't know I'm OK." His
voice is loud.

"I said back off!" Officer Manor yells. She marches into the nursing
station. "This guy needs medication, now. He's threatening me!"

Anne looks up from her medication cart and reaches for a syringe.

"Hold on a second," I say, motioning for her to put the syringe
down. She knows that she works for Bellevue, not DOC, that she only

takes orders from a doctor and that we only use shots when there is a real emergency, but I've seen her side with the DOC on more than one occasion.

I turn to Officer Manor. "What did he do?"

She looks at me with venom in her eyes.

"You saw him. He can't stay in his room. He keeps coming up to me; he tried to grab me. You got to get him some medicine. You hear me?"

I walk a little closer to Officer Manor, feeling less afraid now, like a mama grizzly protecting her cub.

"Yeah, I hear you, but I doubt he needs medicine. Did he actually hurt you?"

"No, but you know he's gonna! He's crazy just like everyone else here."

My face is red and I'm trying to hold my tongue.

"Let me go talk to him."

"Forget the talking; just get him the meds!"

"No," I say more firmly. "You're going to have to wait. And you have to get out of the nursing station." As a clinical space, the nursing station is off-limits to the officers.

She rolls her eyes, not moving. Anne and Luke stare at us.

As if on cue, the veteran Officer Brown steps in.

"Hey, Manor, come on out. Let the Doc talk to him. No need to get into it."

He puts his arms on Manor and guides her out of the nursing station. She is calmer with him around. I follow behind and head to Kevin's room. Manuel is still in the phone alcove, talking as if nothing has happened.

Kevin has closed his door by then. I open it to find him picking at his wrists with his fingernails, digging in and trying to make himself bleed.

"Hey, hey, how about you stop that?" I ask quickly, breaking the rule against entering a patient's room alone. I reach out to him just short of touching. Two nursing techs, one I've never seen before and Alex, a muscular man from Grenada who works as many double shifts as possible to take care of his wife and young children, are suddenly next to me, and then next to Kevin, gently holding his hands at his side so that he can't hurt himself. Kevin doesn't resist.

"Hey, Kevin, it's me, it's Dr. Ford; we met earlier." He has a glassy, unfocused stare, like he's off in another world.

"It's OK, Kevin. She didn't mean all . . ."

"He needs the needle!" Officer Manor yells from the doorway, interrupting me.

I whip around and snarl back, "Will you get out of here, please? You aren't helping the situation."

"That ain't my job," she mutters and walks away.

Kevin is more upset about his phone call than about what Officer Manor said to him. I head back into the hallway to clear my own head, and see a crowd of officers by the nursing station, one of them wearing the white shirt of a captain's uniform. It looks like Officer Manor is being interrogated.

The captain peels off when she sees me come out of Kevin's room. I don't know the captains as well, since they aren't in the unit as much.

"Dr. Ford, let's talk about this," she says, motioning me away from the crowd.

"Sure," I respond, happy for a quieter place to talk and a person to talk to who isn't Officer Manor. I take a deep breath and stand up tall.

"We have a sixteen-year-old patient who's never been here before and desperately wants to call his mom to tell her he's all right. I think he's really sick, but he won't talk to me until he's made that call." Then I relate my version of the events. "Officer Manor completely provoked him," I explain. "She is the reason he started cutting himself in the first place."

"She said that the inmate threatened her first," says the captain. "She said he was about to hit her."

I roll my eyes. "Hardly. He was just asking for the phone. He might have been annoying, but he never threatened her."

The captain nods and looks out the window at the officers still gathered in the hallway.

"Well, what do you want to do?" she asks. "Is the inmate injured?"

"No, he's OK," I say. "I just want to get him on the phone and be done with this."

The captain nods again and heads back into the hallway. She joins the officers and directs everyone but Manor to get back to their posts. I can hear Manor's voice raised but can't make out what she is saying. She points at me a few times as I pretend to be looking through patient charts. Then the captain returns.

"I'm putting Manor on meal relief for the rest of the afternoon" is all she says, and walks off the unit.

Officer Brown is now on phone patrol, and Kevin eventually gets to speak with his mom. When he hangs up, he keeps his end of the bargain and tells me a little more about what happened at Rikers. Kevin says that he talked back to an officer at ARDC who had, in turn, coerced a few of the other inmates to beat him up in an alcove away from the eyes of the security cameras. I am shocked to hear such a horrible story and feels helpless to do anything about it. I'm too new in the job to know the answer to the latter question.

Within an hour, the unit settles back down to the usual routine, with patients pacing up and down the hallway, and therapists and nurses running groups, talking to patients, or writing notes in the nursing station. At 3:00 p.m., a band of DOC officers and a captain do count—they go in each room and make sure that all the patients are still in the unit and that no one has escaped. Nobody mentions what happened earlier with Officer Manor except Alex, one of the techs who had helped hold Kevin's hands to keep him from hurting himself.

"You did the right thing, Doc," he whispers as we pass in the hallway.

Maybe so, I think, but the "A" post officer doesn't make eye contact or say good night as I leave the unit that night.

The next morning, I stand in front of Gate 7, the entrance to 19

North, for an extra-long time. I can't figure out the delay; there isn't anyone waiting at any of the other gates.

"On 7," I finally yell down the hallway to the control room.

A few more minutes go by. It's just me standing there alone in an empty hallway, but I can see the top of the "A" post officer's head, and I can hear the distant hum of radio noise in the control room.

"On 7," I yell louder. Still no response.

I walk down the hall and peer in through the 19 West gates.

"Hi, hello," I call, waving my arms to get the attention of the control room officers. There are two officers in there, both with their backs turned.

"Hello!"

No one turns around, but I hear the 19 North gates slide open. I race back down the hallway and slip in with a nurse.

"Were you waiting there long?" I ask.

"No, they were pretty fast this morning," she says with a smile. "It's nice when it works out that way."

The "A" officer appears at the blue door and opens it with a smile for the nurse. When he sees me, his smile turns to a scowl. Get into it with one of them, you get into it with them all.

7

PUSHING THE LIMIT

I head from Bellevue to my small private practice on the Upper East Side of Manhattan a few evenings a week. I had left the space I'd occupied with Ella and now share an office, a converted apartment on the twelfth floor of a high rise, with Marc. He and I have adjoining offices, but I never see him here. If I'm with patients, then he's home with our son.

I like the quiet up here. Although I still feel awkward and out of place in my private practice, it's a nice contrast to 19 North. I am the only one with the key to my office. No waiting for anyone else to open the door for me. There is a large, comfortable chair in the corner near the window with a view of the East River. There are no bars on the windows.

My patients sit on a black leather couch at a respectable distance across the carpeted room, some clutching one of the throw pillows as they speak, others unsure of whether they are supposed to lie down or just sit as they would in a living room.

"Whatever makes you most comfortable," I always say.

There are a few boxes of tissues strategically placed around the office, a desk where I keep my files, and several framed posters from the NYC subway line—my favorite a drawing by Peter Sís that depicts Manhattan as a giant whale. There's also a closet in my office where I hide all evidence of my personal life from my patients—a trunk filled with bedding, a high chair that won't fit into our one-bedroom apartment already crowded with baby stuff, and a pair of running shoes and workout clothes in case I need to blow off some steam along the river.

I see about ten patients a week, all for forty-five minutes. I don't participate in any insurance plans and I charge anywhere from $50 to $200 a session, depending on what each patient can afford. The illnesses I treat in that office are not all that different from those at Bellevue—I have a few patients with schizophrenia, a few with bipolar disorder, a handful with depression and anxiety—but the issues that my private patients face are wildly different. They have a place to live, a job; many have insurance, and many are women. They are mostly white and mostly rich.

Tonight I am listening to a patient talk about her latest conversation with her mother while I stifle a yawn from the combined exhaustion of my own new motherhood and running the unit on 19 North. I am easily distracted by the fatigue. While my twenty-eight-year-old patient describes how she still feels like a child, I'm thinking of the cooler of breast milk in the closet and how, earlier today, I hurriedly walked by a Bellevue patient post-pump and heard him grunt from his room, "Hey, gorgeous, you a lawyer?"

If I looked like a lawyer, it was the unwashed, disheveled, barely employable kind of lawyer. I clip-clopped down the hallway in my doctor's clogs and an ill-fitting blazer a few sizes too small. I gave up on makeup and contact lenses months before. I hadn't washed my hair in days, but it was up in a bun, so who could tell? There was dog hair and a spit-up stain on my slacks.

"No," I told him, keeping my eyes mostly focused ahead of me. I had other things to do. "I'm one of the doctors here."

"You the head doc?" he asked. His voice was low and gruff.

"Sort of," I chuckled, turning to face him. "I'm the head doctor out of two—does that count?"

He was standing just inside his room, facing the wall and half hidden behind the door. He stared at me with a slight smile on his lips. I could see his right arm moving rhythmically up and down.

"Are you OK?" I asked. Maybe he had some kind of tic disorder or partial seizure. He looked a little out of it.

"Just stand there," he said. "I ain't seen a good-lookin' woman in a while."

"What do you mean . . ." I started to ask, first thinking that he must be crazy to find me good-looking, then quickly stopping myself when I realized what was happening.

"Are you masturbating?" I exclaimed.

I expected that the patients would get excited about a few of the psychologists who sometimes wear high heels and tight skirts, but a flabby lady in mismatched clothes?

"Seriously?" I asked aloud. I was too shocked to be offended. He smiled and nodded his head. He didn't stop and I didn't move. I was stuck to the floor in the middle of the hallway, looking right at him. What is the proper etiquette when you see a patient masturbating in front of you? It didn't seem right to scold him. He was in his room, after all. He was being honest, even if it wasn't pleasant or friendly. I couldn't be angry about honesty. I didn't call for help or run away. I couldn't figure out what to do, so I just stood there and stared back at him. Like looking at a picture that you can't quite understand. Eventually, he stopped rubbing himself and retired to his bed with a sigh.

"That ain't right," a female officer said, coming up behind me and pointing angrily in the direction of the patient. "He can't just do that when you're walking by." She pointed at me. "You should have made him stop."

"Why?" I asked. "He wasn't hurting me. He was just horny. Better he do it in his room than the hallway, right?"

"You just lettin' him play you," she responded. "You really OK with being his jerk-off girl?"

I was taken aback. Not so much by the abrupt language, but by the idea that I might actually be OK with what she was proposing. I wasn't OK a few years before, when a radiology tech positioned my gowned self in a compromising position for a hip X-ray and said, "We sure don't get attractive patients like you in here every day." I was not OK when a drunk correctional officer tried to kiss me at the annual holiday party. I was definitely not OK when, five months pregnant as a new attending and getting ready to testify in the mental health court at Bellevue, the clerk of the court commented on the size of my breasts. Was I really OK with a patient masturbating in front of me? The answer was surprisingly easy.

"He's not attacking me," I replied. "He's not hurting me. He's just being himself and . . ." I stopped talking as the officer turned away and brushed me off with a wave of her hand.

"You got to show them who's in control," she said snidely. "You let them do shit like this and all hell will break loose." She walked off.

" . . . You know what I mean?" my private patient asks, returning me to my cozy Upper East Side office. I tilt my head in a gesture that I hope encourages her to continue with her train of thought and doesn't reveal my lack of attention. Our session ends, but I know I haven't given my patient her money's worth of my time. Within a few months, after many more sessions during which my mind is at Bellevue, I shutter my private practice.

8

WHAT DOESN'T BREAK YOU

I am next up on the "see and advise" rotation—a list of eight psychiatrists and psychologists who take turns evaluating patients fresh off the bus from Rikers Island. Betty, the den mother of the forensic psychiatry administrative staff, interrupts me at three o'clock one afternoon with the message that I am required to head over to intake to do the next evaluation. "All I know is that he sliced an officer with a shank that he whittled out of a toothbrush handle," she says, giving me the one-liner about the patient.

"Oh, great," I sigh. "And I've got to get out of here today by five to get my son from daycare. Let me guess. Is this patient named Peter?"

"Sure is," she replies. "You know him?"

"Yeah. I do."

"You want me to get someone else to see him?" she asks, hearing an edge in my voice. "Gotta think about that baby. The one you're picking up and the one on the way." I'm four months pregnant with baby number two, and have already grown a nice-size bump.

"That's OK, Betty. I'd rather just get it out of the way."

Officer Nelson greets me at the sally port with a booming and friendly, "Hey, Dr. Ford. How ya doin'?" I grin back at him. I have warm feelings for Officer Nelson and most of the other steady officers. Enough

71

days of "How ya doin'?" on a regular basis, and I have started to actually care about how *they* are doing. I think they are starting to care a little about me as well.

I hear Peter before I see him.

"Hey, you over there, shut up so I can think!" he yells loudly from his intake cell. I can also faintly hear another patient rapping about sex with aliens. He must be the target of Peter's vitriol.

"Can't you get him to shut up?" Peter whines. I've made it to Gate 3, just before the hallway that leads to 19 South, the forensic medical-surgical service. The individual intake pens for all the "psychs" look out on this hallway. I can see Peter's ESU officers leaning against the hallway wall with their arms crossed, shaking their heads dismissively at Peter's complaining. They don't see me just yet.

Three years after I first met Peter in this same holding area, he is now perhaps the most difficult and well-known patient incarcerated at Rikers Island. He has been in and out of the jail for more than half of his thirty-one years.

Peter has become infamous during his time in the box. He has racked up more than 800 days of punitive segregation, mostly for assaults, but also for serious acts of self-injury, like cutting his wrists with loose screws from door hinges and swallowing forks and batteries. He is like a caged animal when he gets out for his one hour of exercise—all of his pent-up frustration and rage lets loose on whichever unlucky officer escorts him outside. In the twisted world of jail, where there isn't much to be proud of, Peter contends for the honor of most feared inmate.

Rikers Island sends Peter to Bellevue every so often so that the jail staff can get a break from him. He is definitely sick, but he doesn't fall neatly into any diagnostic category. It is hard to figure out where he belongs in the system. The jail thinks he is too "behaviorally dysregulated" and suicidal to stay there; the doctors at the hospital usually think that he is too manipulative and aggressive to be here.

During an admission to 19 West, about six months before, he

apparently made it a few days before he was found with a shank under his mattress. He used it to cut his arms, and threatened to kill himself if his doctor sent him back to Rikers Island. Even that wasn't enough to keep him in the hospital. The discharge summary read, "He has been evaluated and admitted multiple times, and his behavior has never been seen to be a function of a major mental illness." This is code language for "We don't understand him, so we can't treat him."

Psychiatric hospital admissions are a largely subjective endeavor in New York State, especially when the patient is in jail. The legal paperwork that can force someone in against his will mentions "alleged mental illness" and "likelihood to result in serious harm." Patients who want to be in the hospital, and can sign in voluntarily, need to have a "mental illness for which care and treatment in a hospital are appropriate." None of these terms is clearly defined in the accompanying statutes, so local hospital customs dictate who gets in and out.

Patients who present with clear and classic "major mental illness"—schizophrenia, bipolar disorder, major depression—typically get admitted and stay until their acute symptoms subside, about two to four weeks. Some patients stay longer because we are worried about what might happen to them when they go back to Rikers Island. It's not the same discharge plan as leaving a regular hospital unit and heading home to your family.

Patients without classic mental-illness patterns, patients who are a complicated mix of pathology and learned behavior, patients who are aggressive for reasons that are not easily obvious (like paranoia)—all are hard to treat. There are no medication algorithms, no behavioral plans, no quick fixes. Doctors don't like to fail, and they don't like to feel helpless. So someone like Peter, who can make even the most dedicated doctor eventually feel like a helpless failure, is rarely welcome on an inpatient unit.

The scariest thing about Peter is that he is fearless. "No one can do anything to me that would make my life any more miserable than it already is," he told me the last time I saw him. I kept him longer than usual that time so I could work out an arrangement with a psychologist at Rikers Island to see him three times a week and focus on very in-the-moment skills for him, like thinking twice before he starts yelling an obscenity at an officer. The therapy and the attention worked for a while, but Peter had a huge outburst the day after the psychologist went on vacation, and he ended up back at Bellevue.

This afternoon, he continues to complain about the patient in the adjoining cell.

"All his talking and I can't think straight! Can't you just medicate him or something?" Peter asks the ESU again.

"Maybe the doc can do that," the tallest officer says, spotting me as I come in Gate 3.

Peter sees me and cries, "Dr. Ford, finally! You're the only person in this place I can talk to!"

He's standing up, his wrists cuffed, the fingers of one hand wrapped around the heavy steel bars, the other hand dangling in a clutched fist. He is a wiry, light-skinned black man with deep brown eyes and heavy lashes. I expect to see his long hair but it is gone, replaced by a crew cut.

"What happened to your hair?" I ask first. That hair was Peter's most valuable possession.

"Those motherfuckers shaved it," he says angrily.

"Yeah, when you decided to splash one of us with your own piss," an ESU officer adds from a few feet away. There will be no privacy during this patient encounter. The officers have to stay with Peter, he has to stay in the cell, and the only way I can talk to him is through the bars.

"Shut up!" growls Peter. "You know I'll throw it."

The officers look at each other.

"What are you talking about?" I ask, worried about all the possible things that could be thrown. *The heavy plastic chair in his cell that he had already tipped on its side? The DOC issue slip-on shoes that he could kick off even with his ankles shackled together? His meal tray?*

"Nothing, Doc, don't worry about it," Peter says calmly.

"Ask him what's in his hand," nudges the ESU. "Just ask him."

I take the bait and ask.

"Seriously, Doc, nothing," says Peter. "Let's just get talkin'."

"Wait, I really should know," I say, leaning closer to the bars trying to inspect his hands. The stench makes my pregnancy nausea even worse.

"Whoa, hold on, Doc!" one of the ESU officers warns. "Don't get that close. He's got a piece of shit in his hand."

I quickly back away and look at Peter. He hangs his head in shame and turns away from the bars. I watch him slowly move to the chair, sit down and tuck himself into a ball.

I take a deep breath through my mouth and square my shoulders.

"OK, let's see," I look around. "Where can I sit?"

The only chairs in the hallway are lined up against the far wall, a bench of three padded seats bolted to the floor. If I sit in one of those chairs, I'll be at a safe distance in case he decides to hurl feces at me, but we'll have to yell at each other across this busy hallway. One of the nurses from 19 South walks by.

"Yo, Doc, hold up. You pregnant again?" Peter asks from his fetal position on the chair.

"Yeah," I chuckle, head over to the bars, and decide that standing there is probably the only option if I want anything like a meaningful discussion with Peter. I start to acclimate to the smell.

"How's the other one doing?" he asks. He is less guarded and quiet. It is like we are chatting in the grocery store.

"He's wonderful, thank you," I say before I have time to wonder how he knows that I have another child. I don't remember taking care of Peter when I was pregnant with my son, but somehow he knows. I am too distracted by the ESU, the 19 South nurses, and Peter himself to worry about what else he might know about me.

"Now can you tell me what's going on?" I ask, pointing at the feces in his hand and changing the subject away from my children. "And will you wash your hands before we have a conversation?"

Peter grins broadly, as though my request is preposterous.

"Nope. But I promise you that it won't get anywhere near you. You got a new life growin'. And plus, you've always been good to me, even when I screw up."

So this is how we start talking. The snickering ESU and a patient being wheeled past in a gurney interrupt us every so often, but before long, a half hour slips by. Peter tells me more of his story, more than I'd ever been able to get out of him or been interested in hearing during his prior admissions.

His mother abandoned him when he was an infant, leaving him with an abusive aunt, and then equally abusive foster-care parents and group homes. He never met his father, although he must have inherited his taste for drugs. Peter started using pot in elementary school and graduated to cheap crack cocaine before dropping out of the 8th grade, his report card filled with suspensions, absences, and failing grades. Everyone, including his aunt, told him he would be a failure.

"That last place, Samaritan Village, or whatever it's called; you know that place?" Peter asks, fast-forwarding a decade. He's referring to the residential treatment center where the judge who was presiding over his last arrest had agreed to send him in lieu of staying in jail.

I nod.

"I liked it. At least for the week I was there. But then I fucked it up real bad."

"What do you mean?"

"They got these sirens going down the block and they were gettin' closer. I thought they were comin' for me. I didn't do nothin' wrong, but they'd probably find something to get me for anyway. So I ran right out the back. And now I'm stuck in here again for violating probation."

"Oh, Peter," I sigh. We sit looking at each other in pensive silence. I have no words that will make either of us feel better. I forget for a moment that this man in front of me has brutally attacked many people, and see only a scared child. I can't medicate away his fear. All I can do is sit with him and listen, and try to help him feel safe.

"Do you understand that you aren't responsible for what happened to you when you were young?" I eventually ask him. "That no child should be treated that way?"

He nods silently, although I don't think he believes me.

"But you are responsible now," I continue. "Everyone in the jail thinks you are a monster; you and I both know that's not true. What if you began to change their minds?"

He nods slowly, deflated at the grueling prospect of trying to turn his lifetime of desperation into a life worth living. Incarceration, and especially solitary confinement, has changed him. His survival skills, so long nurtured in the culture of jail, are hard to override. He tells me that the officer he "shanked" called him a piece of shit.

Peter's eyes start to water. He seems surprised to feel the tears on his cheek.

"Talking about all this stuff makes me cry, Doc," he says gently as he wipes tears on his shoulder. "I ain't done that in a long time." He pauses, then adds quietly, "I bet you are a great mom."

Our moment is interrupted when Officer Morales, a very beefy but mild-mannered officer from intake, pokes his head into the hallway. He's been patient while I've been talking with Peter.

"Doc, you almost done? If he's leaving, the bus is waiting . . ."

"Uh, yeah, hold on," I reply.

"Peter, just a second; I'll be right back." I go into the intake area to talk to Officer Morales and get away from the eavesdropping ESU.

In spite of his pain, I know that I'm not going to admit Peter into the hospital. He isn't psychotic, suicidal, or imminently dangerous. He doesn't have one of those classic "major mental illnesses." He is just carrying feces to protect himself. If I were in his situation, I might do the same.

"I'm not going to admit him," I tell Officer Morales. "But he's still got the feces in his hand and I don't want him to get hurt." Morales and I both know that if Peter so much as motions to throw the shit in the direction of the ESU, he will be tackled so hard that one of his bones will probably break.

Officer Morales is a pretty easygoing guy, but this is too much.

"Doc, seriously, he can't be transported with that in his hands. No way. They won't let him on the bus."

"But he'll go quietly if you let him keep it," I plead.

He thinks for a second. He's probably realizing that if he can get Peter out the door without a fight, then Peter is no longer his problem. Whatever happens on the bus, that's not his business.

"Go talk to him again," he says. "Let me see what I can do."

"Thanks," I say. "Let me know."

I return to Peter. He is now pressing his face against the bars, staring at the floor.

"You know you've got to head back to Rikers Island," I tell him as gently as possible.

He nods, as if he has expected this result all along. The sensitive Peter who had surfaced for a brief moment during our interview is gone.

"I know. I just hope nobody messes with me. I ain't gonna take shit from no one."

I make a last-ditch effort to convince him to wash his hands.

"Come on now, Doc, I can't do that. This is all I've got."

"OK, then just hold on. Maybe I can walk you down to the bus." I'm thinking that no one will hurt Peter if I'm around as a pregnant witness.

"No way, Doc," says one of the ESU officers. "That ain't happening. We'll take care of him." They start suiting up in their bulletproof vests and coming forward toward Peter's cell. Officer Morales comes out of the intake area into the hallway with the keys to the intake pens. This is my cue to leave.

"Good luck, Peter," I say, trying to hide the despair that I feel. I am ashamed that I don't know what else to do to help this man; my power-lessness is too much to bear. I break eye contact and turn away.

He presses his forehead against the bars and takes a deep breath. As I return through Gate 3, I peek back and see Peter lift his head up to meet the ESU. He looks defiant and proud. I imagine that he is steeling himself for whatever awaits him on the Island.

My head is throbbing and my clothes reek. My body feels like it can't hold me up anymore. In my office, I slump into my chair and call the number for the Prison Health Service (PHS) psychiatrist who filled out Peter's referral form. PHS is the contracted vendor, hired to provide healthcare to the inmates in the NYC jail system.

No one picks up after twenty rings; that particular psychiatrist is probably gone for the day and probably only works one shift per week. It seems that most of the psychiatrists on the Island are *per diem* staff. From what I've heard about the working conditions at Rikers Island, I would not want to work there full-time either. No cell phones, no internet, crumbling facilities, no ability to reliably get medication to patients, DOC controlling everything.

I try the PHS on-island administrator instead, a 24/7 operator who routes outside calls to each of the twelve non-hospital facilities. A kind voice answers, but can't tell me exactly whom I should talk to about Peter's return, since we aren't sure of exactly when he will arrive back there. The operator patches me through to the voice mail of the mental health unit chief at GRVC, the George R. Vierno Center, home of the solitary confinement cells on Rikers Island. I leave a message that Peter is on his way back, give a brief synopsis of my assessment—"will do best with a consistent provider, will act out the second he feels disrespected or disempowered, is not psychotic; please make sure he is not injured upon arrival"—and hang up the phone.

I want to rest my head on my desk and take a quick nap, but instead rush to pack up my bag and get home to my son.

The chilly evening air helps propel me along the brick-lined pathway between the housing projects on First and Second Avenue, past a dirty playground used mostly by drug dealers and pumped-up early-morning exercisers. I focus on the sound of my clogs on the sidewalk and the horns of angry drivers battling rush-hour traffic and throngs of pedestrians. Navigating the crowded streets keeps my mind off what might be happening to Peter on his way back to the Island.

That night, I spend extra time with my son, bouncing him on my lap and watching him giggle as he brushes up against my belly. He isn't saying "baby" yet, but he knows something is happening in there. I wrap him in my arms and kiss him all over his chubby cheeks, trying to inhale as much as I can of his sweet softness. When I tuck him in to go to sleep, he holds onto my hand and doesn't want me to leave. I rub his tiny fingers and brush his hair out of his eyes, telling him that he is my "first baby born" and the truest love of my life. I fall asleep on the rug next to his crib, our hands entwined through the bars.

A few hours later, I awake screaming. Something is not right. Is he still breathing? Has someone stolen my child? Did I try to hurt him? I can't find a nightmare in my memory to tie to these irrational fears, only raw and overwhelming panic. It takes close to five minutes to settle my heart rate and rejoin the reality of my peacefully sleeping son. I crawl into my own bed next to Marc and eventually drift back to sleep. It will be years before I sleep through the night again.

9

THE LISTENING CURE

"Don't touch that button!" I warn as Cynthia reaches for the red button that's seductively placed next to Gate 7. She pulls her hand back as if she's been slapped. Cynthia is a third-year medical student doing her psychiatry clinical rotation on the forensic service. Today is day one for her—a sensory overload of gates, rules, red lines, alarms, officers, and very sick patients.

"Oops, sorry," she says, then quickly follows up with, "But how come it says 'Push to Open'?" I like that she is wondering about things that don't make sense. I know a whole world of things that don't make sense inside this gate.

"You *can* push it," I say, but caution her about the risk of annoying the DOC officers. "It's just better to stand here patiently and wait for them to see you. It will happen eventually. I sometimes find this is a good moment to take a few breaths and get my thoughts in order. Kind of like forced meditation."

Cynthia smiles and nods respectfully. I don't think she gets it, but by the end of her six weeks, she will.

She starts to take care of patients with me, only one or two the first week. She sits in rounds and listens to the updates on the patients in the unit. Kareem is back with me for another admission, still frantically producing dozens of pages of his book every day; Franklin, who has a history of suicide attempts and depression, has been a patient of Lukes's for months and is doing well despite facing a twenty-year prison sentence; Emile hasn't been here for very long, but we already know him and his distinctive tics well.

Cynthia is intellectually sharp and eager to please, like most of the NYU students, but she is also exquisitely intuitive. In only the first week, when most students are already asking about evaluation forms and reminding me that they will need some time off near the end of the rotation to study for their exam, Cynthia has found a patient about whom she can't stop thinking. She reminds me why this work is so special.

Her patient is Raheem, a mid-thirties Muslim convert from Staten Island who has been upstate in prison for the last nine years on a drug-sale charge. He's with us, as are a few patients each year, because he is temporarily at Rikers Island while he appeals his sentence. However, his situation is a little different. Raheem is stuck in legal limbo. The laws under which he was originally sentenced (known as the Rockefeller Drug Laws) have been repealed, and he is up for re-sentencing, with any luck to be released with time served. But with paranoid fantasies about the FBI swirling in his head, he does not understand what is going on. Until he does, he cannot be re-sentenced. His schizophrenia is keeping him incarcerated.

Raheem tells Cynthia that she reminds him of the women who kept him company while he was upstate.

"You were able to see women up there?" she asks, incredulous.

"Oh, yeah. Leah, she was the most special. I married her when she was born in 1800."

I see Cynthia's eyes shift as she grasps that Raheem is not describing reality. She looks a little flustered, but I stay quiet and let her figure out what to do.

"Tell me more about Leah," she continues. And so begins the

longest conversation Raheem has ever had with anyone on 19 North. Cynthia sits with him for close to an hour, apparently unperturbed by his rancid body odor.

She is fascinated by Raheem's clinical and legal situations. He is the first schizophrenic patient she has treated. He is also the first person she has met who has spent time in solitary confinement. More than half of Raheem's prison years have been spent in the box because he gets in fights and doesn't shower—and at least once, he set his cell on fire. She is also shocked that a man this sick was sentenced to such a long prison term for selling two ounces of cocaine.

I watch Cynthia absorb this information into her framework of what is right and wrong. She is infuriated, and tells me she is going to call her state senator immediately. I share her outrage, but realize that in the short term, there is little we can do. He is still our patient, I remind her, and unless he says otherwise, we are bound to keep his health information private.

"But his legal case?" she implores. "Can't his lawyer fight for him?"

"Yes, and I'm sure she will." Raheem is fortunate to have caught the attention of one of the most dogged and seasoned legal aid attorneys in the city. "But for now, our job is to treat his schizophrenia."

When Raheem agrees to come out of his room to meet with Cynthia, she tolerates the close, stuffy interview room for as long as he wants. When he doesn't get out of bed, she stands at his doorway and talks to him, telling him about the weather and what's going on in the news, asking questions about how he's doing as well. Cynthia has made a connection. It is this persistent caring, over only three weeks, that leads to something no one has gotten out of Raheem in three years. He takes his first soap shower one morning, and the whole staff rejoices.

10

A MOTHER'S LOVE

The patients keep getting admitted to the service, one to 19 West and then one to 19 North, alternating like clockwork. There is an admission logbook—an old, thick, accounting ledger—that is kept in the office suite during the day and on 19 West overnight. About once a week, the nurses complain to me that we on 19 North have gotten more admissions than 19 West—"How is that fair? We are a smaller unit! We only have two teams instead of three! They are keeping patients longer so they don't have as many free beds"—and then I head dutifully next door to my counterpart on 19 West, and we comb the logbook to look for any funny business.

Most of the time the issue is a DOC separation order, which is a security mandate related to gang affiliation, violence, or even family connection, that requires two patients to be on different units. This messes up the order of admissions and sometimes means that two patients get admitted to one unit back-to-back. It all usually works out in the end; only once did we find that a 19 West nurse had intentionally fudged the logbook to prevent an admission.

Mornings without new admissions are like giant sighs of relief. No new charts to populate with piles of paperwork and orders. No new patient interviews that can sometimes last for hours. Breathing room to try to spend more time with the patients who are already here. The wheels of the admission machine spin quickly on the forensic service. There are only these sixty-eight beds on these two units for all of the thousands of men at Rikers Island who might need help.

This particular morning, there are no sighs of relief. We have three new admissions since the day before, and everyone is feeling close to their limit. I try to be as fair in my assignments as possible, but inevitably, someone is going to be upset. Luke and I spoke before rounds about assignments, and he agreed to take two of the three since he had discharged a few patients the day before and has a strong medical student working with him.

"Here you go," I say at rounds, pushing the two brown mailing envelopes bursting with patient records across the conference table to him.

"Seriously?" I hear the activity therapist on Luke's team whisper to the psychologist. I'm sure she thinks I'm not being fair.

Luke opens the first packet and, as usual, starts reading aloud to the group from the Rikers referral page.

"Twenty-five-year-old African-American male with schizophrenia; has been to Bellevue before; refusing all medication; psychotic, violent. Believes he is white."

"Wait, what is that patient's name?" I ask.

"Steven," says Luke.

"Anything in there about an alias? That history sounds pretty familiar."

Luke shakes out the papers onto the table and his eager medical student helps him sort through to find anything that might help.

"Yeah, here," he says. "Says his aka is Jamel."

"I knew it," I say a bit too triumphantly, considering that Jamel was released from custody not so long ago and promptly arrested again, this time for pushing someone on the sidewalk.

"OK if we switch? I treated him last year."

"No problem," says Luke and he slides the re-stuffed envelope back in my direction.

We hear about the other patients: an Asian man who boarded a bus at Port Authority holding a decapitated head, and a middle-aged white man who tried to hang himself at Rikers Island and spent a week in the ICU before being medically cleared to come to psychiatry. I look at Luke and shrug sheepishly as an apology for having taken the easiest of the three patients.

Jamel, it turns out, is not so easy the second time around. I remember him clearly from the last admission, so I go enthusiastically to his room, expecting that we'll shake hands and pick up where we left off. He growls at me and turns away. He doesn't have the gashes in his skin the way he did a year before, but he still believes as firmly as ever that he is a white man covered in black skin. The officers and the nurse's aides, many of whom are black, initially chuckle whenever Jamel claims he is white: "Come on, Jamel, you're as white as my black shoes."

His insults get worse over the next few days and he starts calling officers "nigger" and "monkey." I have many conversations with the various DOC captains and tour commanders, none of whom ever seem to be the same, about how to manage Jamel. We don't agree. They want him locked in his room all the time, as does some of the clinical staff. Even though his incessant verbal aggression is almost intolerable, I can't ethically—or legally—justify the punishment of seclusion. I talk about his case with Luke, with the 19 West attendings when we go to lunch in the coffee shop on the ground floor, with my own therapist twice a week, and with my boss, the director of Bellevue's forensic psychiatry service. No one knows what to do.

After several weeks, he's still not better. He almost punched one of the nurse's aides in the hallway, and the hospital nursing administration is scrambling to find anyone who will work on 19 North. The director is starting to feel pressure from the head of the hospital to find a solution, so he comes to my office every day—sometimes multiple times a day—to get an update. Nursing staff start calling in sick, and I get wind of possible union action if Jamel isn't removed from the unit.

"We can't work like this," says our outspoken nurse, Marie, on a Tuesday afternoon during an impromptu staff meeting in the nursing station. "Does one of us have to get killed to get anything changed around here?"

I wince at this suggestion.

"Just move him to 19 West," says one of the therapists. I am sure this plan won't work. Everyone is as much at risk over there as they are in 19 North.

"He knows exactly what he's doing," says another nurse. "He's just trying to scare us. He should go back to Rikers Island." The complaints are getting louder and more intense.

"Hold on, everyone," says a booming voice from the back of the nursing station. It's Eric, the gentle, yet giant, nursing tech. Jamel has insulted him multiple times. He commands more respect on the unit than I do.

"You guys remember Jamel from last time? He is really sick; you all know that. Let's think about what we are supposed to do in this unit. We take care of sick people, right? The sickest people in this hospital. The doc is just trying to do that also. You lock this guy in, he's going to get worse. He's already so paranoid."

I am so relieved not to be the focus of the meeting for a brief moment.

"He's not paranoid," says one of the nurses. "He's just antisocial."

"No, he's not; he's sick," I hear from someone else.

"But we can't treat him here. It's too dangerous."

The brief moment is gone.

"OK! OK!" I yell to interrupt the cacophony. The crowded nursing station gets quiet. "We aren't all going to agree, but we at least have to have the same plan. Jamel is not going to be discharged and he is not going to move to 19 West. So what are we going to do to make sure we, including Jamel, are all safe?"

I look around the nursing station and see mostly helpless, dejected, and scared faces. Even Eric, when presented with the concrete question of what we should actually *do*, is stumped.

After a long, slow minute of silence, I try again.

"Who has the best relationship with him?" I ask.

"I don't know why, but he seems to talk to me," says one of the psychologists, hesitantly. She is older, white, and a little grandmotherly. "Maybe I could help?"

"He's never given me any problem," says one of the new Filipino nurses.

With the exception of the hardened few, staff begin to forge a treatment plan that involves rewarding Jamel for good behavior, a consult from a psychopharmacology expert in the hospital, and a renewed sense of hope that we can help.

"We've got to sign out," interrupts Marie in the midst of our preparation. "Our shift is over." She is one of the hardened but seems placated that we have a plan.

"Oh, right, of course," I apologize. "Thanks so much, everyone, for your help. I'll talk to the DOC and let them know what we're thinking."

I leave the nursing station and talk with a few of the officers in the unit. I'm closer to them now than when I began the job. One in particular, Officer Sheldon, seems better able than most to ignore Jamel's racial insults. Sheldon told me a while back that he wanted to go to social work school. I share our plans with these officers, at least as much as I can without violating Jamel's medical privacy.

"Give us a few days," I ask, "and if it doesn't work, we'll figure something else out." Officer Sheldon nods, and his colleagues follow. I hope that they can convince the other officers on the unit to do the same.

"Jamel, you have to stop insulting everyone," I plead with him the next morning. "Whatever you believe, if you keep talking like this, you are going to get yourself hurt." I keep my distance and stand safely in the doorway of his room, although I know that my white skin offers some protection from Jamel's psychosis.

"Doc, I ain't supposed to be here, and you know it. This whole thing, it's a mistake. I got my degrees from Harvard and Princeton, I'm a psychiatrist and a lawyer—you know this ain't right. Someone's spreading lies about me and it's one of those niggers out there." He points into the hallway just as Officer Sheldon passes by. I flinch at his choice of words and put my finger to my mouth, signaling for him to keep his voice down with that kind of language.

"Please, please . . ." he whispers. "You've got to believe me! I'm dying here!" He starts to choke back tears and turns to the wall so I don't see him cry. I stand in the doorway and wonder whether it's the right time to talk about medication. Jamel takes what I'm prescribing because it helps him get a few hours' sleep at night, not because he thinks he is psychotic. Best I can tell, none of the alphabet soup of antipsychotic drugs he's been on has ever helped. I have one more option, a medicine that the experts I spoke with last night all think is the best chance to help Jamel. It's not an easy sell.

Clozapine is the magic wonder drug of psychosis, but also has a very serious side effect. A tiny fraction of patients who take it develop a dangerous reduction in white blood cells. Without that critical defense against infection, a simple cold can turn into pneumonia or sepsis—or even death. The FDA did not approve clozapine until 1989, despite its incredible efficacy against difficult-to-treat schizophrenia. Even with approval, it requires monitoring through a national registry and, at least in the beginning, weekly blood draws to check white blood cell counts. Despite this risk, before it was available in the U.S., some American parents smuggled in the drug from Europe by way of Canada to get the only medicine that could help their children fight the serious and painful mental illness that is schizophrenia.

As I watch Jamel cry, I remember the handful of patients I've treated with clozapine; they all got better. One deeply paranoid woman was able, after years of institutionalization, to finally get a one-bedroom apartment. It also worked for a patient named Delancy, who arrived at Bellevue one early morning, having walked to New York from California, most of the way barefoot. His toes were bloody stumps by the time he arrived at Bellevue, and he was emaciated almost to the point of death. Clozapine was the only drug that finally settled his manic and restless feet.

Jamel will probably not be the hardest to convince about clozapine. I have to sell it to his mother, Sarah, as well.

Her love for him is intense and gripping, like a pit bull. We have spoken a few times on the phone over the previous weeks. Or, more accurately, I returned three of the sixteen messages she left on my machine, all berating me for prescribing her son medication. She knows Jamel is sick, but she doesn't trust doctors. Especially white, female doctors.

"He can't have no sex with those things!" she told me a few times, meaning the drugs. "How's he ever going to give me any grandbabies? He's tired all the time; he gets too fat; he just ain't Jamel anymore. Can't you give him somethin' that fixes his brain and doesn't mess with anything else?"

"I wish," I said. "They all have the potential to mess with something."

Although Jamel, as an adult, is the only one who can formally agree to his medication and treatment, Sarah has been a strong influence since he's been in the hospital. Most of the men I treat either have no family or don't want me to contact them, so I am grateful for mothers like Sarah, who care so deeply for their sons.

"Jamel," I eventually say from the doorway, "I'd like to talk to you about a new medicine. I think it will help."

"Go away," he mutters, no longer crying but just staring out the window. "We can talk about it later."

His response is better than I expected.

"Great!" I say overenthusiastically. "I'll find you later today." I hope that he will choose to stay in his room until then. The less hallway time he has, the better.

That afternoon, I am uncharacteristically nervous for my meeting with Jamel. If he says no to clozapine, I'm going to have to let him deteriorate to the point where I ask a judge to force him to take it. I don't want to wait that long, I don't want him to get worse. It seems like his life may be riding on this conversation.

"Thanks for coming in here," I say as he shuffles into the interview room. I close the door and glance through the glass panel at the officer who is supposed to be watching us. She's talking on her cell phone. I make eye contact and motion to her that we are in the room, but she just keeps chatting.

"How are you feeling?" I ask as we settle ourselves into the plastic chairs, Jamel sitting ramrod-straight with his hands on the table. His steely gaze makes him look nothing like the scared man I saw earlier.

"The same," he says. "When are you going to get me out of here? I want to go back to Rikers. I know you write the orders around here. You sent me back last time."

"Jamel," I begin, "I want to send you back, but you're not well enough. We've got to get you on a medicine that works."

"You don't know what you're talking about, Doc. Are you even a doctor? 'Cause you sure don't know what you're doin'." He starts talking faster and louder. "You think you're better than me, right? You think you know everything, but where did you go to medical school, huh? Bet it wasn't Harvard."

"It wasn't Harvard," I say, hoping to catch him off guard with my honesty.

"I know!" he snarls. "Of course you didn't. I know what kind of tricks you're pulling. All these mind games ain't gonna work. I got my psychology degree and my doctor's degree. I'm a lawyer too, so I can sue your ass if I need to. Just get me out of here. I ain't taking any more of this shit."

"I'm really sorry, Jamel. The only way I can get you out of here is to get you on a medicine that works."

"No way, no way!" he yells, prompting the officer to close up her flip phone and come check on us. I motion for Jamel to sit down so the officer will back away.

"I ain't taking no medicine. Forget it. You'll have to find some other guinea pig."

"What if it helps you sleep better?" I say. "What if it means that you only have to take one medicine?" Jamel had been on so many of them that I can't remember them all. "What if it gets you back to Rikers faster?" I am grasping at anything to at least engage him in a dialogue.

"How's it gonna do that?" he asks, sitting back down and now paying attention.

I start with the good stuff.

"It will definitely help you sleep," I say. "You probably won't have as much trouble with erections as you did on the other pills. You'll just take this medicine and nothing else."

Jamel starts to do some calculus in his head. He doesn't think he has schizophrenia, or any other illness for that matter, but he knows his many doctors over many years think he does. He is probably working the equation in his head about how many doses he'll have to take to get out of the hospital. I don't really care why he takes it at this point. If I can get enough of it in him and he starts to see the difference, he'll eventually want to take it on his own.

"There is one risk that you should know about. It's very rare, and can be serious."

I explain about the blood draws every week, that I will make sure nothing is wrong, that the chance of getting sick is very small. Before I even finish, he gets up and leaves the room, shaking his head and mumbling about how crazy I am.

"Just think about it," I call after him. I sit back down alone in the tiny interview room, staring at the dingy white walls. Did I just blow my last chance with him?

I get back to my office later that day to find a big flashing red "7" on my answering machine. I listen to the messages as I take care of some paperwork, only half paying attention to the digital voices. Then a loud woman's voice comes on the line.

"Dr. Ford, this is Sarah. Jamel told me that you wanted to start him on some medication that could kill him. Are you crazy?! What are you doing, treating my son like that? What kind of doctor are you? Jamel ain't stupid, you know, and we'll sue you if you do anything to hurt him. Do you understand? He don't need no medicine anyway. You just better watch yourself, because if anything happens to him, something is going to happen to you. If you think I don't mean it, just try me." She ends by leaving her phone number, "so we can talk."

Despite my line of work, this is the first threatening phone call I have ever received. Jamel probably called her right after he stormed out of the interview room. Reluctantly, I pick up the phone and dial, listening to each ring like an alarm.

"Hello?" I hear on the other end. Sounds like a teenager.

"Is Sarah there, please?"

"Who's calling?"

"This is Dr. Ford," I reply.

"What do you want?"

"Well, I can only speak with Sarah about that, if she's there. May I please speak with her?" I hear some mumbling in the background and then Sarah gets on the line.

"I ain't talking to you no more. You got some nerve calling me here."

"I'm just returning your call," I say, trying to keep my sarcasm in check.

"You got something useful to say? 'Cause if not, I'm hanging up."

"It sounds from your message like you are upset about the medicine? Maybe we can talk about that?"

"We can't talk about nothing," she says. "Jamel is not taking that medicine. I will not let you poison him like that!"

"I'm not trying to poison him, Sarah," I say quickly. "It probably doesn't seem this way to you, but I'm trying to help him, to give you back the real Jamel. If we don't treat him with this medicine, I'm afraid he's going to be gone forever!"

I can hear the desperation in my voice. I am scared that Jamel might die without the medicine, and Sarah is scared that he might die with it. We go back and forth for a few minutes, each upping the ante in our panic. I tell her that I will go to a judge and force Jamel to take the medication if we can't find another way. This brings on a whole new level of verbal assault, and I begin to tune her out. Looking around my office at the sticky notes and memos I leave myself, my eyes rest on a picture of my infant son taken at Coney Island the previous winter. He is bundled up in my arms as we stand in front of the Atlantic Ocean, his nose and cheeks bright red from the cold wind. He is looking at the camera with his smiling eyes and I am looking at him. He was so fragile then, so innocent. I am lost in that boy in that moment, completely and totally in love. I would do anything to keep him safe.

I tune back in to Sarah and hear her words in a different way. She is just trying to protect her baby.

"Sarah," I interrupt, my voice softer now. "I have a son also. I don't want him ever to be scared and alone like Jamel is now. Can we please try to work this out?"

I feel a pang of regret and a little bit of fear as soon as the words leave my mouth. Have I just played a dirty card, tricking Sarah into seeing me as a mother instead of a doctor? Did I reveal too much about my personal life? Is Sarah going to find out where I live and do something to my son?

There is a pause on the other end of the line. I can hear Sarah breathing, and then I hear her crying.

"I don't want him back in the hospital no more," she finally says, her voice quivering. "I want Jamel back to normal. I been through too much these past years. It's harder and harder each time."

She takes a moment and blows her nose.

"Let me ask you, seriously, do you really think he's gonna get better? Do you really think this medicine is gonna work? 'Cause I don't think I can take another situation like this again."

"I know," I whisper, and pause, then continue. "Sarah, I think the medicine will work this time. I'm not sure he's going to be totally back to normal, but he'll be better. He'll feel better. Maybe he'll stop getting arrested so much."

No response on the other end.

"I just need your support," I continue. "Jamel trusts you more than anyone in the world. If he doesn't have your blessing, then Jamel won't try anything. I don't want to go to the judge. Please, we need you," I beg.

The next day, Jamel asks to see me.

"I'll try it," he says, taking me completely by surprise.

"Really?"

"Yeah, I got it," he says. "Don't tell me all that stuff again or I'll change my mind. But if it doesn't work, I'm not taking any medication ever again. That can be on you, Doc. Deal?"

He offers a fist bump. Fist bumps are a sign of solidarity in jail, a greeting that indicates respect and aggression at the same time. On the prison ward, they have been co-opted by some of the doctors and nurses who don't want to shake hands for fear of spreading germs. I counter with my outstretched hand for a real handshake. Jamel looks confused, like it has been a while since anyone reached out to him like that. We grasp hands.

I start him on clozapine, withdraw my request to the judge, and slowly raise the medication a little each day. He is sleepy at first, but otherwise seems to be doing all right. Within a week, Jamel no longer thinks he is white. Within two weeks, he begins apologizing to officers and spending daily sessions with me. Sarah visits him and then calls my office, this time leaving an entirely different kind of message.

"It's a miracle, Dr. Ford," she sobs. "Thank you. Thank you."

The miracle is short-lived. Within another week, Jamel's white blood cell count starts to drop. It isn't yet in the range where I have to stop the medicine, but it is close. I draw his blood again the next morning; the count has dropped even lower. I get another second opinion from a psychopharmacology expert in the hospital to figure out how I can keep Jamel on this medicine, but his count drops again. I ask the lab to double-check that they have the right sample. I am going to have to stop the clozapine.

Jamel barely lets me get the words out before he yells at me and, again, leaves the room. I think of the answering machine full of curses from Sarah that will be waiting for me.

Jamel catches up to me on my way through the gates and out of the unit. He stops just short of the red line.

"You told me that if I tried the medicine that you'd get me back to Rikers," he says. "I don't want to be here no more and I don't belong in no hospital. You gotta keep your end of the deal."

I stop and turn to him.

"I know we made that deal," I say, making a mental note not to make any more deals. "But you had a bad reaction to the medicine, so we couldn't even give the deal a chance. I can't discharge you until we figure out something else."

"Naw, naw, no way. That wasn't the deal, Doc!" he declares, shaking his finger at me and raising his voice. The guard by the gate looks up from her desk.

"You have to send me back to Rikers now. The deal was that I would try the medication, not that it had to work."

He's right, of course.

"If I discharge you now, you'll be right back here in a few days."

"That's a lie and you know it!" he yells. I back myself closer to the gate, safely inside the red lines.

"Jamel, I can't talk to you like this," I say. "I'm going to go to my office. We'll talk later."

"No way, bitch," he mutters, and then stomps away.

"I've been called that a lot," I joke to the officer, embarrassed that I wasn't able to keep Jamel calm.

I go to lunch with the other psychiatrists from the service, Luke and the three from 19 West, and tell them about having been called a bitch. The unit chief from 19 West, a feisty and opinionated woman with whom I occasionally clash, but always respect, chuckles.

"Ah, Elizabeth, if only you knew the things I've been called. Consider yourself lucky that he chose such a nice word."

The other two 19 West attendings nod in agreement.

"You just have to ignore that stuff," says one. "They don't really mean it."

The next morning, a Friday, I come in to more messages from Sarah. I listen to a few of them and delete the rest. I glance at the bed list sitting on my desk, a one-page cheat sheet created each morning with important information about all of the patients on the unit. At the bottom of the page is a "court list," the names of the patients who left around six that morning to a court hearing; if they return, they won't get back until ten at night. Even though patients like Jamel are hospitalized—most of the time, against their will—they are still entitled to due process of the law. That means that they have a right to defend themselves in a criminal courtroom and then come back to the unit. Clinical staff don't go to court with the patients; we rely on the officers to bring them back safely. This does not always happen. A black eye or a busted lip are not unusual after a trip to court. I hear from patients that the real risk is from fellow inmates in the holding pens at the courthouse.

Sometimes I hold a patient back from court if I think that the sixteen hours outside of the hospital will be too risky for his health. I try to reserve this for the very sick, since every missed court date usually means another month in jail while the judge finds another hearing date. No one should be in jail longer than absolutely necessary. If a patient is so suicidal that he will look for a spare piece of shoelace or torn T-shirt to hang himself from an exposed pipe when nobody is looking—that is the man I will hold back from court.

Jamel's next court date is on Monday, so I figure that we'll do the risk assessment about court today in rounds. He is not suicidal, so I can't justify keeping him from his hearing, but he is charged with a low-grade felony that might be bumped down to a misdemeanor. If that happens and he takes a plea, he'll probably be released with time served. The question at rounds will be how worried we are if Jamel gets back out on the street. And then I see it. Jamel's name is on the court list. I cross my fingers that this is an error and call John, the elder caseworker with the rap sheets and legal information.

"Why is he at court?" I ask before he can say hello.

"Who?" John asks.

"Jamel," I say, frustrated that he can't read my mind. "He was supposed to go to court on Monday, not today."

"Let me see," he says. I hear him logging onto the computer and rifling through some papers.

"Hmm, I don't see anything. Sometimes the lawyers schedule additional dates and they don't get loaded into the system. Maybe this is some kind of psych evaluation for the court? Could be a lot of things."

"Is he going to get released?" I ask anxiously.

"Highly unlikely," John replies. "I don't think you have too much to worry about. Looks like he has open warrants and it's a felony charge."

For a caseworker, John is a pretty good therapist. He is soothing and calm in a way that is contagious. I hang up the phone and stretch out my tense shoulders, relieved that I don't have to worry about what Jamel might be doing out in the world. I sign out to the evening psychiatrist to check on Jamel when he comes back from court that night and to expect that he will be upset. Jamel probably thinks he's getting released that day. I leave orders for extra medicine just in case, but I hear nothing all weekend.

When I return to the hospital on Monday, Jamel is gone. He was released from court on Friday after taking a plea.

Since I didn't know he was scheduled for court, I hadn't sent a letter to the judge explaining that Jamel was on a civil commitment hold. That is a legal status whereby he is kept in the hospital against his will because he is—as confirmed by three psychiatrists and as a result of mental illness—"likely to cause serious harm to himself or others." Instead, he is now out there somewhere with no medication, no phone numbers for any doctors, and no documentation that he has ever been hospitalized at Bellevue.

I go into crisis mode. My heart starts racing, my muscles start tightening, and my mind clears itself of whatever cobwebs were floating around in there. I call Sarah, the court administration, John, the shelters, and the police. I try unsuccessfully to reach the judge who released him. I call ERs in the city and colleagues at other hospitals. I put out an APB over the psychiatric community airwaves, but get nothing in response. He has disappeared.

For the next several days, until a new crisis arises on the unit, I look over my shoulder as I walk to and from the subway. Six months along with my pregnancy, I wrap my hands around my belly like a protective belt. I scan the headlines of the *Post* and the *Daily News*, expecting to see something about a crazy man released from Bellevue. I tell Marc about Jamel—not because I want him to comfort me, but because I want him to take extra care with our son when he picks him up from daycare. I jump and easily startle and worry. Remembering Jamel's final words to me—"No way, bitch"—I am actually scared.

11

EVEN THE STARS CAN FALL

I am like many female physicians who have young children—trying to avoid the gnawing feeling of inadequacy that comes with taking care of children and patients who need so much. My adult patients seem to become virtual children when they lose their autonomy in jail. If I take some extra time to read a story to my son in the morning, it is at the expense of my patients and colleagues. At the end of the day, if a patient, perhaps unsettled by being locked up, needs my attention, I come home late to a fussy son and a weary husband.

Well into the second trimester of my pregnancy with a baby girl, it is hitting me hard. The all-day morning sickness and swollen ankles are uncomfortable, but the comments and the looks from the female officers, especially Officer Manor, are worse.

"You shouldn't be coming to work, Doc," she says derisively. "It ain't safe." I feel simultaneously shamed and proud by her words. I want to stay on the job just to prove her wrong.

The men are much more sensitive, like Officer Brown.

"You need me to walk with you?" he says. "Want me to stand by the door?" he asks when I go to interview a patient. I don't want to be treated any differently than Luke or the psychiatrists on 19 West, but the pregnancy has made that impossible. The hormonal pool in which I'm swimming has also, I think, started to mess with my head.

I cry most nights recalling the stories I hear all day of patients' childhoods, filled with abuse and neglect. I snap too easily at the nurses, especially Marie, when they speak sharply to the patients. I have trouble discharging my patients to Rikers Island because it feels like sending them to a dungeon. I can only see the pain and suffering that my patients have endured, not the pain and suffering that they have inflicted on others. Once, in the middle of rounds, I begin to think about a patient who'd told me that he was locked in a closet for several days when he was three years old. I can't stop the tears, and have to leave the room.

I publicly blame the pregnancy hormones, although I know my emotional dysregulation has much deeper roots. Luke, ever gracious, takes over running the unit for that day while I see my other patients and write notes. I am grateful that for one day, I don't have to think about our bed capacity, the leaking ceiling in Room 30, or the stats about length of stay that are due to my director in a few days.

On one occasion, I have to treat a patient accused of creating infant pornography. I can barely get through his assessment. His crime is an integral part of his illness and I can't ignore it, but I hold my breath and count silently to twenty as he details how easy it is to photograph naked children being raped. I focus on the numbers and the sound of my voice in my head so that I can block out what he's saying. I am starting to practice dissociation—the ability to mentally distance oneself from a situation—in order to survive. If the counting doesn't work, I allow my eyes to glaze over and let my thoughts drift elsewhere.

After he finishes, after he tells me about having been raped over and over by his mother's boyfriend, he begins to weep. This is when I am no longer able to hold onto my dissociative trance. His emotional intensity bleeds over into my own. I feel the outrage at what he does to these children replaced by pity and empathy. He is sending these images over the internet, he says, because the customers who covet them make him feel important. They praise him for his artistic style and appreciate the prompt delivery of his product. He craves this validation, this love.

Sometimes it seems anything can drive me to tears. Newspaper headlines, for example: "Boy Killed as Overloaded Van Hits Pole on Harlem River Drive," "Teenager Accused of Murder," "2-Year-Old Left in Car Overnight." I ask Marc to screen *The New York Times* and clip out stories that might trigger my panic. Only a year into my leadership on 19 North, despite couples therapy, in part triggered by my ambitious career choice, Marc and I struggle to stay connected. I no longer talk to him about my patients or my work. I have no interest in being touched, and startle when he puts his hand on my shoulder. One night, he forgets to double-bolt the door in our doorman-protected, security-patrolled neighborhood. I rage at him and he is relieved to see that I can at least express emotion. In the middle of the night, when I wake from a nightmare, he reaches his arm out to soothe me and I swat him away.

The work, however, continues. One chilly day in March, Marie calls my office.

"Can you come into the conference room?" she asks. It is an unusual request.

I arrive a few minutes later to find the head nurse sitting next to Marie and Alex, the kind nursing tech who had helped me with Kevin and Officer Manor the year before. All three of their heads are down.

"What's going on?" I ask.

"Show her," Marie prods Alex in her thick Caribbean accent. "She has to read it."

Alex pushes a handwritten statement in my direction.

"I gave this to the police a little while ago," he says. "They said they were going to investigate."

The words I read unfold like a bad dream.

I was approached in an aggressive and intimidating manner at an intersection in Brooklyn by Jamel X. He came very close up to me, close up to my

face and within striking distance, and said to me, "Do you remember what I
told you at the hospital? Remember I told you that I would bust a cap in you
when I see [you] on the streets?" I answered yes. He then said, "You're lucky
this time, 'cause the next time I see you, you're going to get it."

"Oh, my God!" I exclaim and turn to Alex. "Are you OK?"

"Yes, yes, of course," he answers, "but I called the cops. He shouldn't
be out there on the streets."

"You did the right thing," I assure him. "Is it OK if we let the other
staff know? Just in case they see him?"

Alex nods.

A few more minutes pass while Marie berates me, the judicial system, Bellevue, and anyone else she can think of about having let Jamel
leave the court. Eventually, she simmers down and returns to the unit
to make assignments for the evening shift. Alex feels safe enough to
head home.

I wait about a week for Jamel to get re-admitted to Bellevue or to
show up on WebCrims, the public website that lists everyone arrested in
New York City. He doesn't come back. I look for his name in the papers;
nothing there either. I check in with Alex every day, but he gets tired
of my hovering and asks me to stop. Marie quickly redirects her complaints from the courts back to the Bellevue nursing administration. On
the surface, everything seems back to normal.

12

WHEN DARKNESS COMES

"I don't think I can do this anymore," I tell Marc one night over a dinner of takeout chicken and mashed potatoes. My son sits on my lap and plays with the Bellevue ID card hanging from a breakaway lanyard around my neck. "And with this little one on the way," I say as I point to my large belly, "it's only going to get worse."

"Well, do you want to quit?" he asks bluntly. He knows that I am not happy, and while it will be hard, he can probably support us with his income from private practice.

"No, not yet," I tell him. "But I'm going to give up the unit chief job." He looks relieved.

I talk to the director the next day and tell him my plan. I don't think he knows what to do with a pregnant woman in tears sitting in his office. He lets me blubber it all out and then—very matter-of-factly, just like Marc—assures me that it's no problem. Luke can be the unit chief, and I'll just be a regular attending. Responsible only for my twelve patients, and no one else.

"Thanks so much," I tell him. "I think this will really help me be a better doctor."

I talk to Luke a few days later after the director presents him with the unit chief position and he accepts. I can't tell whether he is excited or not, but I offer to help out as much as I can. We arrange for a transfer date a few weeks away, and when that Friday arrives, I gladly inform the staff that they can page Luke with any problems overnight or on the weekends. It is a massive relief to cross my number off the call sheet.

The next Monday, early in the morning, one of the 19 North patients hangs himself from the gates at the back of the "L" hallway. It is Franklin, the patient who had been on the unit for over six months, coping with major depression and anxiety after having been sentenced to twenty years in prison. It appears that he calculated when the techs come by for their fifteen-minute checks, found a window of time in the middle of the night when no one was looking, and ran to the end of the hall, tied a sheet around the bars and his neck, and let his weight drop. An officer found him, called for help, and immediately cut him down. Franklin was intubated and taken to the ICU, but he had essentially no brain function left.

I don't learn of Franklin's hanging until morning rounds. Luke wasn't called when it happened either. The charge nurse giving the report describes the events with little emotion or detail. I think she is scared that someone might be fired. One of the psychology students looks like she is in complete shock, and has to rest her head on the conference room table. Only days before, Franklin was playing checkers and Ping-Pong with the other patients, coming to group therapy, and taking his medication. I, too, feel shocked. I had never been this close to a suicide attempt before.

Luke and I work together to organize plans for the rest of the day—checking on Franklin in the ICU; a community meeting to debrief with the patients; a similar meeting for the staff; a review of Franklin's medical chart; staff interviews to find out how this might have happened and implement whatever quick fixes we can identify; and a meeting with our director, the man who will bear the brunt of the administrative pressure from hospital leadership. He is fair and measured in his response, asking only that we start preparing a report and keep him informed of every

SOMETIMES AMAZING THINGS HAPPEN

new development. I am close to tears, and he seems careful not to push me over the edge.

I visit Franklin in the ICU and listen to the rhythmic swoosh of his ventilator. His family—people I did not know existed until then—greet me and are oddly understanding about the situation. I wonder what Franklin has told them that he didn't tell us. He hadn't allowed anyone to call his family while he was in the hospital.

Within days, Franklin is dead.

I am technically no longer the unit chief, Franklin was technically not my patient, and, over the course of the lengthy investigation that follows, no lapse in care is identified. But I feel completely responsible for his death and for the grieving patients and staff left in its wake.

Franklin's roommate, who knew him for only a few days, feels immense guilt to the point of being almost suicidal himself. He says that he heard Franklin rustling around in the middle of the night but didn't think it was anything serious. He didn't want to get into Franklin's business. That's normal around here; almost everyone sticks to themselves so they won't be victimized or be called a snitch. Friendships, camaraderie, attachments—those are fleeting and dangerous.

Some of the other patients in the unit seem almost unaffected. The ones who have been locked up for a long time have seen this kind of thing before. Suicide is the single leading cause of death in American jails.[1]

---

1 Department of Justice, Bureau of Justice Statistics, *Mortality in Local Jails and State Prisons, 2000–2013—Statistical Tables*, August 2015; http://www.bjs.gov/content/pub/pdf/mljsp0013st.pdf

13

SHELTER THE BROKEN

"Elizabeth, can you pick up Eaton?" asks Luke during rounds in one of his first weeks as unit chief. He knows that I don't want to take the other patient, a heroin addict arrested for shaking his ten-month-old baby to death. After having become a mother, and especially after having treated the infant pornographer, I made a deal with Luke that I will not treat patients who are accused of serious child abuse offenses. "It is as much for their sake as mine," I rationalized to him. I cannot guarantee that I will always make decisions that are in those patients' best interests.

"Sure," I reply. I'm still thinking about Franklin and hoping that Eaton is merely psychotic and not suicidal. I read from his chart and learn that he is aggressive and doesn't like to talk.

Morning rounds wrap up, and I join John, the caseworker and only member of my team available for an admission interview, to go see Eaton. According to the bed list, he's supposed to be in Room 27, one of the high observation rooms across from the nursing station. There are no patients in the back hallway near the bars where Franklin tied his sheet. The DOC installed fine wire mesh over the bars and visibility mirrors on the ceiling; there is also a 24-hour watch at the mouth of the hallway, but those rooms remain empty for now. Even if they were open, Eaton, as a new admission, would still likely be placed close to the nurses' station.

We approach his doorway and see an edgy white guy pacing around and talking to himself.

"Eaton?" I ask. This man doesn't look like the patient described in rounds. He looks up and makes brief eye contact, but keeps the loose associations flowing out of his mouth.

"You do not have enough tissues for my issues. I have a big Scooby-Doo and they don't have a clue. Spoonful of sugar makes the happiness go round. I check myself before I disrespect myself. Too much information, TMI, which will give you TWB, teeny weeny bladder, laughing at me, one flew over the cuckoo's nest."

I can't stop a smile spreading over my face and hope that this is Eaton. His brain is coming up with some amazing connections. I need to get the medical student in here to listen.

"Eaton?" I ask again. This time he shakes his head in the midst of his rhyming psychosis and points at the giant lump on the far bed. My smile fades. Eaton is going to be less fun than this other guy.

John and I walk slowly into the room and assess the blanket-covered body. The only sign of life is a slight rise in his chest.

"Should we wake him up?" I whisper to John.

"Wake him up, don't shake him up, break him up into pieces of gold and silver. The silver lining in the gray cloud . . ." Eaton's roommate riffs.

John shrugs his crooked shoulders and offers no advice.

"OK, let's see what happens," I say.

I walk to the edge of the bed. "Eaton?" I ask for the third time. No response. I say his name a little louder. The lump moves.

We spend the next few minutes in a futile back and forth trying to coax the blanket off Eaton's head. It's too risky to pull it off ourselves. Let sleeping giants lie. We leave him and make a plan to return within a few hours.

The few hours arrive in about fifteen minutes. I'm talking to another patient in one of the interview rooms and hear "Crisis Management

Team!" blare over the loudspeaker. I poke my head out and see a tall black man wearing pajama pants on the floor in the hallway, in front of the high observation area. He is struggling with two officers.

"I'm sorry—can we talk a bit later?" I ask my patient, directing him out of the room and walking toward the commotion as quickly as my pregnant self will allow.

"Get the fuck off me!" the patient on the floor yells. "I can't breathe! Get the hell off me!"

The officers are on their knees, struggling to handcuff the patient's wrists and shackle his ankles so that he can't punch and kick. There are grunts and curses flying, but I can't exactly make out whether they are coming from the patient, the officers, or both. One of the officers has beads of sweat lining his brow and is breathing heavily. One nurse stands in the hallway, but everyone else seems to be watching the take-down from the safety of the nursing station. Reinforcements arrive in the form of two more officers, who pick up the patient—face down—by his arms and legs. There is no more struggling; movement is difficult in this hog-tied position.

A crowd including John, me, a medical student, and Alex stares at the scene. I do nothing as the officers take the patient off the unit to the intake area. I'm not supposed to go back there during an "extraction," and I don't even try. Once the patient is out of the unit, I join the rest of the group in the nursing station.

Marie starts telling me what happened.

"He wouldn't get up for the search," she says, referring to the daily random DOC hunts for contraband. "So they picked him up out of bed and yelled and put him against the wall. He started yelling back, and then all of a sudden, everyone was on the floor."

"Who is the patient?" I ask.

"Eaton," she says. I am dismayed but not surprised.

"Did he throw any punches?" I ask.

"Not that I saw, but you never know."

Eaton returns to the unit about an hour later. John and I try to engage him again in an interview. He is sitting in his bed, awake and talking, but I can't track what he's saying. I mostly just listen, because every time I try to ask about his symptoms or history, he cuts me off and continues in his paranoid narrative. I turn to John to see whether he has any questions for Eaton. He shakes his head. We extricate ourselves from the interview we tried so hard to organize, arrange to come back separately later in the day, and head out of the unit. I've seen dozens of patients like Eaton before and am pretty sure that once he sees me a few times he'll start talking.

Back in my office, Captain Tejada, a mid-level boss in the DOC, arrives with paper in hand.

"Doc, you got to fill this in," she says, somewhat apologetically, and presents me with the familiar legal-size document. It is a clearance form asking for my assessment of whether Eaton is safe to go to solitary confinement. I like Captain Tejada. She seems to understand the issues we all face on the prison ward, trying to reconcile the conflict between treatment and punishment.

"What's the infraction for?" I ask.

"He resisted the search," she replies.

"You know what I'm going to do, right?" I ask.

She nods. "I'll come pick it up before the end of my shift."

The first question on the clearance form asks for my determination about Eaton's guilt and whether he should be punished. I am in no position to judge this—and don't want to—so I leave that section blank. The second question presumes that he is guilty and asks where he should serve his punishment: the CPSU (Central Punitive Segregation Unit) or MHAUII.

I don't check either option, willfully resisting the instructions on the form. Instead, I write, "Eaton is currently hospitalized for an acute psychiatric illness." I hope that this simple statement will make both this form and Eaton's solitary confinement go away.

Captain Tejada arrives back just before 2:30 p.m., and scans the form.

"You know those docs at Rikers will complete the form as soon as he goes back to the Island, right?" Captain Tejada tells me. There is no malice in her voice, just indifference. "Whatever you do or don't do, eventually he'll wind up in the box. It's only a matter of time."

Captain Tejada's words hit hard, highlighting my growing sense of powerlessness and utter frustration. I can help patients get better on 19 North, but then what? The DOC escort them out of the hospital and they are gone, out of my control. Those who return to Rikers Island may not see a doctor or get their medication for days, lost in the mass of humanity churning through the chronically understaffed jail. Whatever ability I might have at Bellevue to shelter my patients from this giant, incomprehensible, and trauma-inducing system quickly disappears as soon as they step on those freight elevators and head to the ground floor.

Those who are released from custody are at least free, but then what? Many of them are still sick and get transferred to one of the civilian psychiatric units at Bellevue, where they are stigmatized with labels—often misguided—like "antisocial," "malingerer," and "violent criminal." I get complaints that "my" patients are taking up beds for people who really need them, as if incarceration somehow negates a lifetime of serious mental illness. The message I hear is that forensic patients are less worthy of care and that maybe, by association, I too am less worthy as a doctor.

14

UNRAVELING

The more men I treat, many of whom are coming back on their second or third admission, the more I begin to question what I'm doing. If it's true, as Captain Tejada said, that regardless of what I do my patients are going to wind up back at Rikers Island in the same crappy situation that got them admitted to the hospital in the first place, then what am I trying to do? Why am I fighting, if the outcome is just going to be the same?

By now, I am seven months pregnant and seem to experience life to a heightened degree. I start to have disturbing dreams about my son, dreams that often involve dismemberment or kidnapping—leftover images and feelings from patient stories I've heard that day or the day before. And yet, even knowing this, the dreams seem real. I start to mirror my patients' emotions, crying with their depression and laughing with their mania. I have lost my ability to either filter or contain their sentiments. I am no longer a stable presence in their midst. Most of all, I can feel my simmering anger starting to boil. I cannot soothe myself, think on the bright side, or see the big picture. My patients are starting to become a burden, just a bunch of people I have to see in order to write my notes and go home for the day.

I don't share this with anyone at work, but they must know. Everyone in my field is familiar with the psychological toll this kind of high-demand, low-control work can take. We share an unspoken connection, each experiencing the trauma and the mission of the forensic service in our own unique, but shared, way. Luke probably notices my withdrawal first, but he is too polite to bring it up. I gradually stop going by the offices of my colleagues for a quick venting session, preferring instead to plow through my work and be gone as quickly as possible at the end of the day. I close my door more often and block everyone out.

I know that my passion for the work is starting to fade. I assume it is related to the impossible balance so many working mothers try to find in their lives. Every day I tell myself that it will pass. I become absorbed with Eaton's case; this reassures me that I am still devoted to my work. Some days he is lucid and obnoxious, prompting people like Marie or Bradley, the primary psychologist in the unit, to call for his speedy discharge. On other days, he speaks to the voices in his head and is clearly absorbed in some alternate reality. Sometimes he yells and threatens other patients or staff, but he doesn't hit anyone. He takes his medication about half the time—long enough that a judge will never agree to force him to take more, but not long enough to make a meaningful difference in his psychosis. He still doesn't get along with the officers, but after that DOC extraction a few weeks before, he never again refuses a search.

Then, one week in the late spring, a month before my daughter is born, it becomes clear that even my interest in Eaton's pathology cannot overcome my growing fear, one that's been masquerading as ennui.

The Tuesday of that week starts quietly enough. I have a light schedule with only one meeting. The most recent busload of admissions, weekend transfers from Rikers, was tucked in the day before. I meet with my team after rounds, interview our newest patient, and check my to-do list for the rest of the day. The faster I can check off those little boxes, the faster I can get out of there.

One of my tasks is to write a second opinion on whether a patient, Clancy, should be medicated against his wishes. Keith—the psychiatrist taking care of Clancy—has decided that he is too sick to go without medicine and does not have the ability to accept or decline treatment. In New York State, when a hospitalized psychiatric patient, even a prisoner, refuses treatment he clearly needs, a judge, using more than one doctor's opinion, is petitioned to decide on the matter.

I waddle over to 19 West to evaluate Clancy. I treated him for several months the year before and I think I know what to expect. He is hearing voices. Whatever the voices are saying, they are making him angry with his doctors. He rarely speaks, withdrawing more and more into those voices, and I anticipate that he'll refuse to speak to me as well. But he surprises me by getting out of bed as I approach and agrees to come to an interview room. As we walk down the hall, trailed by the court-appointed Mental Hygiene Legal Service (MHLS) attorney who is required to represent Clancy in the court proceeding about his medication, Clancy glances down at my belly.

"This is your second, right?" he says.

I am shocked at his recall and wonder how this man, so psychotic, can remember such a detail. Not long before, one of my patients who had been hospitalized twice—once during each of my pregnancies—thought I'd been pregnant for eighteen straight months. It seems that my large belly is memorable.

We sit down in one of the interview rooms, short and narrow chambers with a table in the middle and doors at either end. The attorney goes through the usual disclaimers, emphasizing that she only represents Clancy on the medication issue and not on his criminal case. Patients often confuse the two and think that the medication hearing is somehow linked to getting them out of jail. Clancy seems to understand, so I launch into my questions.

"Why aren't you taking your medicine, Clancy?"

"Let me show you," he says. "You take ten pills"—here he mimes taking medication—"then you drink some water."

He points to his stomach and begins yelling, "Don't take the medication! Don't take the medication!" Again and again he points to his stomach. I ask him why he is doing this, and mimic his actions by pointing at my own abdomen. At once, I realize that I have made a terrible mistake by drawing attention to my pregnancy. Clancy jumps up so fast his chair goes flying back behind him. He shakes his fist at me and moves toward the door.

I am half in his way and struggle to get myself out of the chair. He pushes past me and stomps down the hallway to his room, cursing my unborn child with every step. His attorney looks at me, terrified. I try to be cool.

"Well, I guess that answers the question about whether he needs medication or not."

I reach down with some effort, right the chair, and leave the room.

The attorney trails behind me and whispers, "That was scary."

I act as if the event is routine, but as we head back to the nursing station, I admit to the attorney that I'd erred in pointing to my belly, knowing that the most psychotic patients are the ones most likely to respond in unpredictable ways to my pregnancies. Cartwright, for instance, was a man who always screamed wild curses at me from his doorway. Two months before, however, he began to come out of his room and stomp around the unit as I checked on the patients. Each day he inched a little closer, until eventually we were walking side by side—as if he were my bodyguard. He said nothing, but it was clear that he had appointed himself to watch over me. Clancy, it seems, is having the opposite reaction.

By Wednesday, I begin to question whether working with violent patients is worth the risk. I gather my team to accompany me to a meeting with a schizophrenic patient named Simmons. His jumbled thoughts and foul personal hygiene aren't improving. He'll have brief moments of lucidity, but most of the time, I can find no logic in what he is saying. Sometimes his behavior is so outrageous—I saw the man talking to his socks—that he seems to be faking. But he isn't faking, and his brain is getting progressively more disorganized. His neurotransmitters are like faulty electrical circuits.

The interview room is small for all of us. I stand leaning against the back wall while the others sit at the table. At first, it seems as if we might have a rational discussion with Simmons. He knows our names and is able to talk about his medication and about a criminal court hearing he is scheduled to attend. Then, all at once, he interrupts the conversation and asks if I want to sit down. I thank him, tell him I am actually more comfortable standing, but ask if he prefers I sit for the rest of the session.

"Pregnant ladies shouldn't stand," he says with emphasis. "You really should sit down."

Then, without warning, he pops up, grabs the plastic chair he's been sitting on, holds it aloft and throws it in my direction. It goes flying over the head of the psychologist, who has ducked, and crashes into the wall. A correction officer and Eric, who is standing outside, rush in to make sure we are OK.

"Whoa, Simmons, what are you doing? You can't throw chairs in here!" Eric yells.

"I was just offering her my chair," Simmons says, timidly. "No pregnant lady should stand while other people are sitting."

"Thank you," I reply, trying to hide my panic and also keep Eric and the officer from removing Simmons to the quiet room, a padded cell off the hallway for patients who need the psychiatric equivalent of a "timeout." If he has to go in there, we won't be able to interview him again until later, and I don't want to wait.

"Maybe," I say to Simmons as calmly as I can, "that wasn't the best way to make the offer?"

Then he sits back down and picks up the conversation as if nothing has happened. We try to get him to talk about his behavior, to apologize, but in truth, my heart isn't in it. I am, for the first time, thinking almost entirely about my unborn child and not much at all about my patient. I care little for Simmons.

15

BURNOUT STRIKES

Ray is lying in the far bed, up against the grated window. It's gray and cold outside, and the view of the U.N. building is obscured by sheets of rain. A soft neck collar, the kind worn after whiplash, is around his neck. A thin sheet covers the rest of him. A temporary nurse's aide who's covering for Alex (out on worker's comp after breaking his finger trying to restrain a patient) stands outside the room, ordered to watch Ray wherever he goes. Ray was found hanging in his punitive segregation cell at Rikers. He was immediately cut down and taken, unconscious, to Elmhurst Hospital in Queens, the nearest emergency room to the Island. He was there for weeks, slowly recovering from his neck fracture and suicide attempt. When he no longer needed round-the-clock medical care, he was transferred to us. He looks like a sick man who should be in a hospital, but I just want him out.

I don't have proof yet, but I know Ray is responsible for the matches that turned up in a few of the patient rooms during the search earlier today. He's got them stashed in his neck collar. No one wants to take the collar off to check, because every time they get too close, he threatens to swing. He forced an elderly patient to give him his breakfast one morning. He's been insulting the staff and provoking the officers. On my way down the hall, I overhear an officer mutter something about wishing Ray had just died at Rikers. Bradley, the psychologist, doesn't think Ray really wanted to die. He thinks he was just trying to get out of the box and got carried away. I have been trying to meet with him for a few days, but so far he's refused all of my offers to help. I'm annoyed with him.

The unit has been pretty quiet today. Ray has stayed mostly to himself, and we don't have any new admissions. I am hoping to leave a little early and treat myself to an acupressure foot massage. My feet no longer fit into any of my shoes.

I briefly introduce myself to the nurse's aide and ask, "How's he doing?"

"Same, I guess." The aide doesn't seem very interested.

Ray rolls over at the sound of my voice.

"What do you want?" he sneers.

"Come on, Ray, I'm just checking on you. You haven't talked to me since you got here. I'm trying to help."

"You want to help me? Then get the hell out of my room!" he yells.

I'm tired of trying to get this man to engage in his life, and now I'm itching for a fight. I'm not thinking about my swollen ankles any more.

"I'm not leaving," I say tersely. "I'm your doctor and I'm trying to take care of you."

"You ain't tryin' to do shit," he says. "I ain't talkin' to you."

Then the words that I try never to say come spilling out of my mouth.

"If you don't let me help you, there's no reason for you to be in this hospital. I'll just send you back to Rikers."

His defiant glare is intense.

"You think I'm not gonna do it? You think I won't kill myself? Just send me back then; go ahead, 'cause I promise you that this will be the last time you ever see me alive."

He's pushed me too far. I'm already so close to the edge that all I need is a little shove. I no longer feel scared that he might kill himself. I am no longer interested in trying to help him find hope. I no longer care whether he lives or dies. If he wants to play chicken with me, he can go ahead, I think. I've worked too hard to take care of people no one else wants. Maybe I'm done with taking care of souls that other people have broken.

"OK, then," I say, my face red with anger. "There's nothing else I can do. I'm not going to let you blackmail me into keeping you in the hospital."

Ray's helpless pain can't even awaken my empathy. I turn to go and shrug my shoulders at the aide, who now seems very interested.

"I'm done," I say. "Make sure to watch him closely. He might try to do something."

I want to grab Ray and scream. I want to demand that he take some responsibility. I want him to own his problems, to grow up, to act like the thirty-five-year-old man that he is. At least I have the sense to get myself out of the room.

I feel as helpless as he does. Despite my years of training and experience working with men just like Ray, I still don't know how to get through to him. I don't know how to convince him to trust me. I don't know how to earn his respect. I don't know how to turn this patient into someone who has not had the life that he's had. I think I've lost all hope.

That night, asleep on the floor next to my son's toddler bed, an old recurring nightmare visits me again. I used to have it regularly when I was a child, but it had been decades. In the dream, I am on the sidewalk next to my childhood home, and I'm being chased by something. I don't know what it is, but I am terrified and need to get away from it as quickly as possible. I try to run, but my legs are like lead weights; I can barely pick my feet off the ground. I pump my arms as fast as I can, trying to get enough momentum to hurl the rest of my body forward. I get my legs going a little faster, but it's like running through heavy molasses. Whatever is chasing me is getting closer, and I can do nothing about it. I think I am going to die.

I wake up whimpering and sweaty. For a moment, I'm not sure where I am. Then my son's soft snoring brings me back to reality. I am temporarily soothed, knowing that he and I are both safe, but the anxiety and fear quickly set in again. I move to my own bed, hoping to be calmed by the presence of my sleeping husband. It doesn't work, and I lie awake through the anxious hours until daylight.

Ray is the first topic of discussion at rounds the next morning.

"This guy is a real problem," says Marie. "First, he took off his neck collar and refused to put it back on. Said he didn't need it anymore, since he was going back to Rikers. Then he got the plastic knife from his meal tray and started cutting his arm before the watch could get it out of his hand."

"What was he doing with a plastic knife?" I demand, allowing my frustration with Ray—and, frankly, the entire criminal justice system—to be directed at her. I am as much to blame as anyone. "He's supposed to be on a suicide watch!" Luke doesn't rein me in.

Marie, chastened, looks around the table, hoping someone else will have a response. They all have their eyes averted, no one wanting to lock gazes with me.

"What are we going to do about Ray?" I continue. "Is he talking to anyone? Has he gone to any groups?"

"He is mostly in his bed all day, and then he gets up around dinner," says the activity therapist. "He stuck his tongue out at me the other night; I know he tried to touch one of the other therapists. No one wants to work with him."

"It's true. He is disrespectful and provocative in group. It's all antisocial," Bradley says, referring to antisocial personality disorder, a spectrum of symptoms that includes lying, cheating, stealing, and fighting. "There's nothing Axis I," he continues, referencing the psychiatric classification for acute mental illness. "He's terrorizing the unit and should not be here anymore." Bradley thinks I'm being too lenient, allowing someone without a serious mental illness to remain in the hospital.

In earlier days, I would have politely—or not so politely—reminded Bradley that Ray was struggling, whatever his diagnosis, and that we should do our best to find out how to help him. After all, I would have said, he did almost kill himself. That's serious whether he meant to die or not.

A few months ago, I wouldn't have turned away a patient like Ray. I knew that a sad and desperate life didn't give anyone a free pass to behave badly, but maybe it earned a little tolerance. I hadn't yet met a patient labeled as "antisocial" who didn't have a poignant story to tell. If you listen to the story long enough, you can figure out why these patients behave so badly. Then you can try to fix it.

Sitting at the rounds table, I know I am not going to be able to listen long enough to Ray's story. I am starting to see Ray as others see him—a guy who preys on the weak and manipulates the system. Just another criminal.

Marie startles me out of my thoughts.

"Just send him back to Rikers," she says.

Six heads bob around the table. There is consensus.

"Isn't there anything we can do for him?" I ask, hoping that someone else, anyone, will make up for my lack of empathy. *How about that eager young psychiatrist at the other end of the table, Monica, the forensic psychiatry fellow?* She's in the same place I was a few years before, deciding to work in the unit because she knows she can make a difference. Her head is down and she is silent.

"All right," I concede. "I'll get him on the noon bus."

I think I'll feel guilty about sending him back to Rikers, but instead, I feel relief. Within a few hours, Ray will be someone else's problem.

At my office, I write up Ray's discharge summary, a recounting of his relevant history pre-hospitalization, his treatment and behavior during his admission, and his diagnosis and prognosis. I give him a wimpy Axis I diagnosis—Adjustment Disorder—and then change my mind and slap him with "Antisocial Personality Disorder." I can feel myself punishing

Ray as I doom him to carry that label when he arrives back at the jail. I know that when the doctor sees it, he will assume that everything Ray does, even if he is in serious distress, is a lie. I can try to explain the underlying reasons why he behaves the way he does—and I do—but the doctor will only focus on that damning diagnosis.

One copy of the summary gets faxed over to the mental health service at Rikers, and I walk the signed original, in a sealed envelope, over to DOC intake. The handoff of that envelope is DOC's signal that they can start the process of moving Ray out of the unit, back into his orange jumpsuit and shackles, down the DOC-only elevator, out the secluded back entrance of the hospital, onto the Department of Correction school bus, and into another much more dangerous intake area at AMKC. Ray may sit in those cramped and overheated intake pens for days before being placed in a more stable housing area.

I am not allowed, per DOC security policy, to tell Ray, or any patient admitted to the service, that he is being discharged. The DOC does not want inmates to be able to plan for contraband exchanges, gang assaults, or escape attempts. It is, perhaps, the most counter-therapeutic rule in the unit, because planning for transitions and next steps is a critical component of psychotherapy. Symptoms get worse with the unexpected.

I walk the discharge summary over to Officer Morales, silently asking myself whether this is going to be the last one I submit.

"Finally," Officer Morales chuckles when he sees the name. "I was wondering when you guys would get sick of Ray."

I smile weakly and walk away.

16

OUT OF THE DEPTHS

The decision to quit is easier than I think. After almost two years of trying to be a good mother and a good doctor, sometimes failing at both, I choose my children over my patients. One month before my daughter's due date, her estimated size is creeping up to the level of my son's, who weighed in at more than ten pounds at birth and broke his collarbone squishing his shoulders into this world. My OB strongly recommends that I "take it easy" in this final stretch. It is a natural transition to start my maternity leave early. I avoid any uncomfortable discussions with the director, convincing myself that I may change my mind about quitting once I get a real break from the service.

I should really take an extra week to say goodbye to my patients, provide some closure for them, and gradually introduce them to their new doctor. But I just want out. I can't wait. Another week on this service and maybe another patient will throw a chair at me.

I prepare a written sign-out for Luke with all of the important details and to-dos for my eleven patients. In spite of my burnout, I still have a soft spot for Eaton. I am sure he is schizophrenic, which makes him, in my eyes, more vulnerable and less responsible than someone like Ray. But at times, his normal mid-twenties self regresses to teenage behavior in this strict yet unpredictable environment, and he breaks out with foul language when he is angry or foot-stomping when he doesn't get what he wants. This doesn't match everyone's notion of what a schizophrenic should be. So most afternoons, I get a request to please discharge Eaton. I ask Luke to pay special attention to him, so he doesn't get sent to Rikers Island the day after I leave.

Saying goodbye to the staff is quick and efficient; they expect to see me in a few months, cooing about my next newborn and closing my office door to pump breast milk at lunchtime.

I pack up my office the following evening with the assistance of my eighteen-month-old son watching from his stroller and my husband lugging heavy boxes of books to the service elevator. I am mostly relieved at no longer being responsible for patients' lives. But mixed in with that relief, just under the surface of consciousness, is massive grief.

17

DEATH AND BIRTH

All I can see are rooftops and sun reflecting off the skyscraper windows. A few lonely but well-tended penthouse trees wave in the late spring breeze. I come up here to the rooftop garden of my apartment building, five blocks east of Central Park, on most days in the weeks since I left Bellevue. The garden is vibrant with life, and at the same time so serene—quite the opposite of 19 North. I have found peace up here for the first time in many months, although with only a few weeks before my delivery due date, I am feeling slightly less peaceful.

Today, the air is crisp and clean, but I can't seem to catch my breath. The logical explanation is that it's the pressure of my enormous belly pushing against my diaphragm, but I know it isn't that. I have just spoken with Marcy, one of the 19 West psychiatrists who moved over to 19 North in my absence, and my central nervous system is fully reactivated.

Earlier in the morning, the phone rang as I was thinking about what to pack in my baby bag for my trip to labor and delivery. Bellevue's main number flashed on the screen. Thinking of my years of late-night pages and interrupted family activities made my shoulders tighten. *Let them leave a message*, I thought. *I'm done with Bellevue for a while.*

Later on, I checked my messages and heard Marcy's voice.

"Hi, Elizabeth," she said with an uncharacteristically somber tone.

"Really sorry to bother you at home, but hoping you can give me a call at some point. Something's happened here and you should probably know." She closed with a half-hearted, "Hope you are having a restful time off."

I called her back immediately. We spent a few minutes catching up with small-talk pleasantries.

Then she paused, and started again. "Remember Eaton? The patient you signed out to Luke?"

"Yeah, of course," I interrupted. "I hope he's still there."

"Well, no," Marcy answered cautiously. "He died a few days ago."

"What do you mean?" I stammered. I can't understand what she is saying.

"We don't know exactly what happened," Marcy continued. She described preliminary reports that there had been a fight with the DOC, and maybe Eaton had grabbed a walkie-talkie and hit an officer, or maybe worse. There had been an extraction. The DOC called an emergency in the intake pens because Eaton wasn't looking so well, and Luke was the first to arrive. He started CPR; the hospital code team arrived within minutes, passing through the gates opened wide so that there would be no delay. Not long after, Eaton was pronounced dead.

Waves of nausea washed over me when I heard this news. Tears started to flood my eyes. My brain was spinning. My grip on the phone tightened and I let out a whimper. My baby girl started kicking inside. Marcy had no idea what to say, but she kept talking, and her words were somehow soothing.

"I thought you should know. He was here a while and you took care of him for most of that time. I'm so sorry."

I cried and sniffled for a little longer while she kindly stayed on the phone. Then my confusion and grief turned to anger.

"Was there trauma?" I asked. "Was there blood?"

"I don't know," Marcy replied. She didn't offer any explanations or assumptions. She was good that way, never taking a side or spreading gossip.

I had a hundred more questions. Marcy wasn't going to answer any of them. I thanked her for the call and hung up. It was only my pregnancy that kept me from screaming and smashing the wall. Shock, fear, confusion. I felt all of those things. But mostly I felt blinding, helpless rage. Not exactly about the loss of Eaton—about him I felt mostly sorrow—but about what I imagined was an awful death.

Now, on the roof garden trying to find some solace, I struggle to catch my breath. Eaton is on my mind continuously. I think about him as I finish packing my baby bag; I think about him when I pick up my son from daycare later that day; I even think about him when I dream that night. In one dream, I am running through quicksand to save an unidentified man. In another, I watch my son score the winning soccer goal, only to be kicked in the head by the goalie. A crowd of celebrating teammates and coaches initially hides my unconscious son from view, but then I see his fluorescent green cleats poking out of the scrum. I wake up in the midst of sprinting across the field. This is too much for me.

I only make it through a few more days before I call Luke to get more details. I didn't want to call him—I suspect that he is more devastated than anyone else in the hospital—but I can't hold off any longer.

Luke is strangely calm when I call. He is probably still in shock. He doesn't tell me much other than that both the DOC and the hospital are launching independent and huge investigations. I hang up feeling even more adrift.

Within a week, my daughter is born and I forget about Eaton.

As my maternity leave draws to an end, I still can't face the thought of going back to the nineteenth floor. I call the director and tell him I'm not returning. I accept a part-time job in the psychiatric emergency room, three days a week, 8:30 a.m. to 4:30 p.m.—no overnight call, no pagers, no responsibility. Compared to 19 North, this sounds like a walk in the park.

18

REUNION

The alarm goes off at 4:00 a.m. I am an early riser and my three-month-old daughter is not sleeping for more than four hours in a row, but I have yet to get used to this wake-up time. It's hard on the mind and body, right when cortisol levels are dipping and slow-wave sleep is setting in again. Everything is quiet, almost dead, at that hour. This black calm is exactly what I need—the only time of the day when I do not have a child, a husband, a patient, or a boss demanding my attention. Sometimes I go for a run around the Central Park reservoir. It's dark and spooky then, but there are enough hardcore New Yorkers doing the same thing, so I don't feel particularly unsafe. Sometimes I do yoga in the alcove next to the kitchen, as far away from the kids' room as possible. Eventually, I'll find a pool that opens at 5:00 a.m. and head there. Sometimes my body is so tired that I just sit and stare out the window. It is the solitude I love. The solitude I need. Without it, I am what my children will later euphemistically refer to as "grumpy mama."

My time in the CPEP, this mommy-friendly part-time work, is not as restful as I expected it would be. I feel like a visitor every time I arrive for rounds, usually late from the same whirlwind daycare drop-off I managed while in 19 North. I don't know these nurses, doctors, and social workers there the way I know Marie, Anne, Eric, John, and Luke. I miss them and all of the difficult situations we endured together, almost like a family.

I mostly supervise the first- and second-year residents as they interview the new arrivals and decide whether the patients need to be admitted upstairs to the psychiatry units. The work is very fast-paced and I almost never see the same patient on a Thursday that I saw on a Tuesday. The patients come in and out, night and day, psychotic, violent, and suicidal.

There is one group of patients that I do enjoy—the patients brought in by the cops, under arrest but not yet arraigned. They usually arrive handcuffed and shackled to wheelchairs under escort of two police officers, exactly as I remember from my intern year. Except now, I have the authority to treat them the way I want. I can decide to take a few extra minutes to call their family for information; I can sit with them and offer advice without an attending rapping on the window, telling me to hurry up.

I am the honorary NYPD psychiatrist on the days I am there. I try to instill in the residents an understanding of the very complicated interface between mental health and criminal justice. For example, coming to the hospital doesn't get anyone out of jail. In fact, it just prolongs the time to arraignment, when an arrestee sees the judge, gets a lawyer, and begins working on the case. Without arraignment, no one gets released. One patient waited two months to be arraigned on a misdemeanor charge that carried a maximum sentence of fifteen days.

When I explain this situation to the patients, they pretty quickly fall into two categories—those who suddenly realize that they aren't as sick as they thought, and those who are so sick that they don't care. The latter group interests me the most. They remind me of the patients I left behind on the nineteenth floor.

One day, while reviewing a discharge note on an NYPD case in the cramped space of the CPEP, I see Kareem's unmistakable figure through the window, carrying around pages of the same book that he has been writing for years. I scanned and did not understand thirty-seven of those stained pages last year. Kareem is yelling at Byron, a tech I remember from my internship—the one who resembles a teddy bear with his over-sized beige scrubs, squat but very sturdy frame, and brilliant smile. Others are starting to gather around. I see a nurse head into the medication room, nestled in the central office area out of reach of any patient, just in case one of the doctors orders a shot of medicine to keep Kareem from hitting anyone. Everyone is tense.

I head out onto the main floor to join the crowd, inappropriately joyful for the occasion.

"Kareem!" I say loudly. "Hey, Kareem!"

Byron turns around and motions me away. I ignore him. Kareem and I make eye contact and we both break out in broad grins. I raise my arms as if to hug him and then remember where I am. I lower my arms and offer my hand instead.

"Hey, Dr. Ford," he smiles. "What you doin' down here? Will you please tell all these losers that I'm not going to hurt them? They need to calm the hell down."

Byron and the nurse behind me bristle.

I chuckle. "No, I won't tell them," I say. "You tell them."

"What do you think I've been saying?" he starts to yell. "They don't listen!"

"Dr. Ford, let us manage this situation," says Byron. "He can't just be yelling like this."

"What 'situation'?" demands Kareem, pointing at Byron's chest and then his own. "You mean me?"

"Whoa, hold on," I say to no one in particular. Then I look directly at Kareem.

"Come on. Do you want everyone to be scared of you? No one will listen to you the way you are yelling. Why don't we just go in there"—I point toward an interview room—"and talk?"

"Tell them to stop getting the needle ready," he says. "They know it's illegal to give me that if I'm not dangerous to myself or others." Kareem has been in and out of hospitals so many times that he has the lingo down. "And plus, I'll sue your asses."

"OK, OK," I say, holding up my arms in submission. "No needles."

Byron and the nurse shake their heads and mutter under their breaths. Several other techs have now gathered, but they slowly drift away as Kareem and I head into the interview room. I can hear them talking about how I don't respect them or the work they do. "Just another doctor who thinks she knows everything. Kareem's going to talk to her, and she'll think she's made such a big difference, and then he'll punch one of us," I hear them say.

Kareem and I sit in the stale-smelling interview room for close to an hour, reminiscing as though we were old buddies. He told me that he started smoking crack as soon as he was released from jail and got picked up two days later for menacing someone on the subway. The NYPD did him a huge favor and decided not to arrest him, so he came in as an "EDP"—an emotionally disturbed person. EDPs are patients whom the cops could arrest but don't because they are so clearly mentally ill.

Kareem is too delusional in his belief that he is in charge of the CIA to be troubled much by his situation in the CPEP. He believes that as soon as he gets access to his cell phone again, he can call his security detail to come get him. The reality is that Kareem has been homeless for years, in and out of jails and hospitals. I admit him again, to one of the civilian units on the eighteenth floor, and he goes upstairs without a struggle. He'll eventually be discharged to the men's shelter up the block, no less delusional, but no longer yelling at people.

19

BACK TO THE FIRE

I've finally started to be able to read the newspaper again. I can look at a front-page photo of devastation in some faraway land and not be overcome by breathtaking terror. I still can't watch movies that even hint at child abuse, but at least I have graduated from fluffy romance comedies to a few action-adventure films. I'm calmer. I've almost slept through the night at least once in the previous two weeks.

One warm Tuesday in June, the CPEP is particularly slow. There are no overnight referrals waiting to be seen, and everyone who is being admitted has already been assigned a bed and gone upstairs to a unit. Someone has left a copy of *The Village Voice* on the desk by one of the workstations. I pick it up and begin absentmindedly leafing through the articles about a protest at Union Square and the return of Hugh Jackman to the Broadway stage.

I come upon a story that brings my mind back into sharp focus. The article describes the death of a patient, almost a year before, on the Bellevue forensic service. I start to feel a little queasy. The reporter writes about a walkie-talkie.

Wait a second. Wait . . . this is familiar. The walkie-talkie. This sounds like Eaton, but the reporter is talking about someone with a different name. My breathing increases and my heart rate spikes. I look away from the article to slow myself down. Then I continue on, a few paragraphs down, to read that while the autopsy report listed the decedent's cause of death as "undetermined," his body had evidence of fresh bruises and internal bleeding.

This is about Eaton. It must be. I get online at home as soon as I can and read through the *Voice* article again, as well as anything else I can find. A lawsuit was filed in federal court against the Department of Correction, this must be why the death became public.

I stare at the screen in silence as my two children crawl and toddle around the apartment. I should be screaming or crying, but the fear, anxiety, and rage from two years before are nowhere to be found. Instead, I feel a deep sense of calm that Eaton's death is no longer a secret.

The article comes shortly before I hear of rumblings up on the nineteenth floor. A new doctor is hired and then fired four days later. Another doctor is too afraid of the patients to talk to them. Daniel, the friendly and very bright CPEP director, occasionally returns from Bellevue leadership meetings; he reports, when we meet for supervision, about the friction between the forensic psychiatry service and the rest of the psychiatry department. There's always drama up there, I tell him.

Then, in the winter of 2009, the director of the forensic psychiatry service, my former boss, leaves. I don't know whether he is fired or fed up, but within a day, he is gone. I call upstairs and check in with Luke to see if he has any more information. He and the other psychiatrists up there are just as shocked as everyone else.

Daniel is asked to do double duty and run both the CPEP and the forensic service while a search begins for a replacement. He spends most of his time on the nineteenth floor. Two psychiatrists have left and a third is on his way out. I don't know how they are even admitting patients to 19 North or 19 West anymore; there aren't enough doctors to take care of them. In the previous month, Daniel has changed. He has dark circles under his eyes, his shirt is untucked, and he's put on some weight from too many Chinese takeout meals in his office.

He calls me into that office after my shift one Tuesday for a "chat." I have never had one of these before; it sounds ominous. He asks me to close the door, and I immediately think I am in trouble. I sit on the edge of his threadbare couch and anxiously wait while he finishes up a phone call.

"Hey," he says in his usual easy tone. "How's it going?"

"Ummm, good," I hesitate, then add, "You know, same old stuff."

"Yeah, well, would you consider trying something new?"

"What do you mean?" I ask, confused.

Daniel says he has recommended me for the director position on the forensic psychiatry service, and that he thinks I'll probably be offered the job soon. The director is responsible for both of the inpatient units, 19 West and 19 North, as well as two clinics in the Bronx and Manhattan where patients are evaluated for competence to stand trial, and an outpatient commitment program called Assisted Outpatient Treatment (AOT).

He continues: "You care more than anyone in this hospital about those patients; you know the nineteenth floor up and down; and, frankly, we need to get someone up there soon. I can't keep doing this coverage."

My face turns red and I say, incredulously, "Seriously?"

"Yeah, seriously. You would be great at it."

I can't keep the smile off my face.

Even though I left the forensic service only two years before—and still have a startle response that makes other people jump—I am deeply tempted. The walk along the "L" corridor of 19 North is still procedural memory for me. I miss walking through the sally port on 19 West and being greeted by Officer Nelson's "Hey, Dr. Ford!" I think of Eaton, Kevin, and Franklin; I want to build a service where those things don't happen anymore. I want to be the first woman and the first mother to run the forensic psychiatry service.

By the time I meet with the chief of psychiatry, my potential new boss, to discuss the offer, I am ready. I know that I am at risk of becoming angry and cold again, as I was with Ray, although I am better able to take care of myself than I was before. I have a good therapist, a supportive husband, and two kids who turn around my mood the second I see them. When I ask my children, "What is mommy's most important job?" they giggle with glee and shout, "To protect us!" The roots of that answer are buried in my own darkness and fear, but my kids have made it all seem lighter.

I receive Marc's blessing to go back to work full-time. He adjusts his schedule to help more with the pickups and drop-offs at day care. I steel myself to re-enter a world where little is fair and much is beyond my control. In making the decision to return, navigating the pros and cons with Marc, I ask myself the same question over and over again: What will I regret more? Passing up this opportunity in favor of a safer and easier path, or trying to make a real difference? Just as my decision to quit two years before became inescapably clear, so now is my decision to return.

20

WELCOME BACK

My new office on the 19th floor has been empty for over a year. Although this is the office that had been occupied by the director of forensic psychiatry since the "H" building was completed in 1986, my immediate predecessor chose instead to have his office in a newly renovated space, shiny and clean, but farther away from 19 West and 19 North. I am returning to the center of the action.

The dust on the built-in desk that runs the length of one wall is so thick I have to peel it off. There are a handful of screws scattered around the dirty floor, and a rusty filing cabinet leans against one wall. A set of stacking chairs and a Dell desktop computer from the early '00s round out the other pieces of furniture in the room. Along the far wall, there are five built-in lock-and-key cabinets from the '80s, the kind with doors that flip up vertically and are covered with carpet-like upholstery. I lift the lid on one of these cabinets and find two dead cockroaches.

"This place needs a good power-wash," I tell Carol, the new den mother of the forensic psychiatry service. I know her from sometime before this, although I can't remember where or when we worked together and am too embarrassed to ask. She gives me a giant bear hug as though we were best friends. Carol is warm and motherly, but cracks the whip when she sees something she doesn't like.

"Get environmental up here," she calls to the receptionist outside my door. "Dr. Ford's office is a mess."

"No, no, that's OK, it's not a rush," I protest. "Just whenever it can get done."

"Oh no, Dr. Ford, we're going to get this clean. Don't you worry." She hurries out the door and is gone in a whirlwind of energy.

I return the next day, a Saturday, in a rental car driven by Marc and piled high with books, pictures, and diplomas for the walls, a few trinkets, and my two children. They are strapped in their car seats, eager to ride the elevators and see Mommy's new office. Marc parks the car at the back entrance of the hospital while I procure an old gurney for all my stuff. We slowly make our way to the elevators, Marc trying to push the loaded gurney without toppling it over and me holding tightly onto our almost-four-year-old son and two-year-old daughter. The elevator ride doesn't thrill them as much as they thought it would, but the office suite provides plenty of entertainment.

"What's this?" asks my son, pushing all the buttons on the shared fax machine. "And this?" he yells, picking up a stapler. My daughter is happy just toddling around my office while Marc and I quickly unload the gurney into the now clean and polished space. Once my daughter spots the giant whiteboard on one wall and the dry-erase markers resting nearby, she insists on a chair to stand on and sets to work creating what will become the first of many kid-produced murals on that board. My son joins and writes his name in whatever space is not occupied by my daughter's smiley faces.

The remnants of their artwork are still on the whiteboard when the DOC deputy warden in command stops by to say hello the following week. The "Dep" controls the security of the nineteenth floor. He (in this case—occasionally it's a she) manages the fleet of tour commanders, captains, and officers on 19 West, 19 North, and 19 South.

I didn't interact much with the Dep when I was a unit chief, mostly just the captains and officers assigned to 19 North. The director did all of the sensitive negotiations with the Dep around issues like patient and staff safety, investigating bad outcomes like what happened to Franklin and Eaton, and navigating the gray area between health and security. The Deps seem to change every six months as they get promoted up the ranks to supervising warden and beyond. Even though this one just received news that he is on his way up, I am grateful to meet him, and feel for the first time like I am now the director.

Male psychiatrists have always managed these male wards at Bellevue; I am the first woman to head the division. It's May 2009, and the inpatient service is down three psychiatrists. I have my hands full. The chief and I have recruited two who are fresh out of fellowship—Gerald and Kerry—to start after July 1, and I'm working on another to start in October. I will be able to hand Gerald the unit chief position on 19 North once he gets up to speed, but until he and Kerry arrive, I will be the only attending psychiatrist on that unit. I am also now responsible for the rest of the division—19 West, AOT, the court clinics—so, for now, my goal is not to improve the service or make any major changes. I just want to ensure that no one dies.

21

UNDER THE SURFACE

Mental health care comes in two flavors on Rikers Island—general population (GP) and mental observation (MO) units. Those in GP, who have milder symptoms, come to the equivalent of an outpatient clinic in each jail; those on residential MO units typically have serious mental illness and stay on the unit all day. The doctors and therapists come to them.

The MOs are supposed to be the safest houses in the jails, but in reality they are some of the worst. From what I hear, gangs control many of them, immediately threatening the sickest patients into giving up their phone PIN codes and commissary money. The one or two officers who are posted on these locked units are as much at risk of being assaulted as the patients. Clinicians are scared to go inside. There are no nurses around, so a pharmacy tech comes with the medication cart twice a day and dispenses pills through a tiny window in the central control room. Most of the patients don't take their medication.

These MOs are, in part, the reason that about 40 percent of the patients on the Bellevue prison ward have been in the hospital before. They cycle between the hospital and the MOs, getting better in the hospital and then getting worse in the jail. No one knows what to do with these patients.

I've got one now, Emile, the patient with the tics whom I treated when I was unit chief: he's taking up all of my energy. Luckily, I have a bit of relief because the head of the substance abuse division has loaned me one of his fellows—a psychiatrist doing extra training—for the month of June to help take care of the patients on 19 North.

I wish I could give Emile to the fellow, but that would have been cruel to both of them. It will be good for Emile to see a familiar face, even if we haven't always gotten along.

Emile's problems are immense and overwhelming. For every successful admission to Bellevue, he is turned back to Rikers a handful of times, evaluated as not having the "right" kind of diagnosis for hospital treatment. He's not unlike Peter in this way, problematic wherever he goes. He also shares Peter's fearlessness and acute sensitivity to feeling rejected.

"That guy is always fighting," one of the doctors from Rikers Island tells me when I call her to try to get some information on Emile. There is a hint of admiration in her voice. "I saw him once with a punctured lung and he was still swinging."

Emile has been in and out of jail and prison and hospitals for so long that no one remembers what he was like when he first arrived. It isn't until he shows me a picture of himself in the outside world—dressed in crisp jeans with a chain pocket watch and vest—that I believe his claims of being a ladies' man. I only know him as scrappy, dirty, and sick.

Emile is plagued with many things in his life, but perhaps the worst is a neurological disorder that leads to seizures and tics. His tics come with no warning and are not always the same; sometimes he screams "Fuck you" or wags his tongue suggestively during a therapy session. The first time he did this to me, I let out a squeal and jumped out of my chair.

"Sorry," I chuckled when I settled back in. "I've got to get used to that."

"Naw, Doc, no one does," he said. "They never have."

He has genuine and "pseudo" seizures in addition to his tics. Most people think he is faking, but I think his thirty-year-old neurological system is so messed up that his body doesn't know real from fake anymore.

He's never been able to make it through an MRI because the tight tube freaks him out, and the various attempts at 24-hour EEG monitoring have all ended with the wires pulled off his head and an EEG tech cowering in the corner. Emile has never actually hit a clinician before—his targets are officers, other inmates, and himself—but the clinical staff are scared of him nonetheless.

Since there is no scientific evidence of his seizure disorder, and because we can't understand his pathology, many of the staff think that nothing is wrong with him. They think Emile is willfully spitting, cursing, and yelling so he won't get discharged back to Rikers Island.

This entrenched antipathy to Emile surprises me. Something has changed on this unit since I left it only two years before. Bradley seems more wound up than he used to be; Marie is more stubborn and sometimes defies orders; even Eric looks like he's lost some of his enthusiasm. No one seems particularly excited about taking care of patients. I worry that they are as burned out as I was when I left. My first mission is staring right at me around this conference room table during morning rounds—I've got to get people excited about their work again.

Emile becomes part of that mission. I spend close to an hour a day with him, trying to contain all of his complaining, tic-ing, and threats so that they don't disrupt everyone else. He starts to play more Ping-Pong, and that helps keep his muscles in control. I start to do actual therapy with him, working to find something that he wants to talk about, something that he wants to work on. He is a very smart guy underneath all those tangled neurons, and over a few days, he starts to talk more and tic less. It's his pain, emotional and physical, that weighs him down. Pain that no one seems to believe. He tells me that he has to fight to convince people that he hurts.

I know what it feels like to be in pain and have no one believe you. It is humiliating and shameful and makes the pain worse. A few months after I got engaged to Marc, I started having cramps in my right side. They felt deep, somewhere in my pelvis. Sometimes it hurt to walk, but mostly it was an unexpected take-my-breath-away pinch, accompanied by gripping nausea. It must be some weird ovulation pain, I thought, until it went on for a month. My younger cousin had recently been diagnosed with an aggressive brain tumor; one of my friends had just discovered a lump in her breast; and my dad was getting a prostatectomy. I was full of cancer paranoia.

I ended up in the ER at NYU, the same ER where I had spent many nights as the psych consult. They did a serious workup—STD tests, an ultrasound, an abdominal/pelvic CT, lots of blood work—but the only thing that showed up was a small dermoid cyst. I was told it was nothing that should cause the kind of pain I was experiencing, and was referred to a highly regarded gynecologist. When I saw her a few days later, the disdain in her voice was clear.

"It's just not possible that a cyst that small is causing your pain. There's nothing else wrong. I don't need to see you again for this. Maybe it's all in your head."

She didn't believe me; she didn't want to deal with me. She looked at me as if everything I was saying was a lie. I felt completely unheard and trivialized, like I didn't matter.

After some years of therapy and having settled into my marriage, the pain gradually faded away. It was probably, indeed, "in my head." Maybe it was related to marriage and fears about losing my identity. Maybe it was anxiety about becoming a mother. But regardless of why it happened and why it disappeared, that pain was still real to me. And I know that for Emile the same is true.

In the ten days that we work together, Emile gets calmer. He isn't screaming as much and he hasn't had a seizure, fake or otherwise, in a few days. The staff, while still exhausted, seems calmer. As Emile is beginning to get better, I am also getting him ready for discharge. It is a curse of the job that I rarely get the chance to work with patients who are doing well. As soon as one is stable, two more are waiting to get admitted from the Island.

In what is going to be our last session, although I cannot share that with Emile, he brings up a recent fight between two patients.

"I heard one of 'em got hit really bad," says Emile. "That ain't right. No one should be hittin' that hard around here."

"Hmm," I say. "I'm not sure anyone should be hitting at all around here." I try to steer the conversation away from the specifics of the fight.

"Do you feel upset about it?" I ask.

"Hell, yeah," he says. "That kind of stuff makes everyone around here look bad." His voice starts to rise and his right hand starts to tic. He starts talking fast and furious, getting more and more worked up.

"I gotta get out of here, Doc! Let me out of here!"

I get up and fumble with the doorknob trying to open the interview room door. The doorknobs are particularly challenging now that they've been altered. They changed them after a patient looped a sheet around the old knob in his room, tossed the sheet over his door, slammed the door shut, wrapped the sheet around his neck, and used his body weight both to hang himself and prevent anyone from getting in the room. Eric finally pried open the door with a crowbar stored in the nursing station. The patient survived, but the old door handles didn't.

I never really get used to the new ones. They are flush with the door and higher than most handles, angled and tapered so that anything a patient might loop around them in a hanging attempt—a ripped pajama seam, a torn bed sheet, soggy toilet paper coiled into twine—will slip off. I apologize to Emile as my hand keeps sliding off the doorknob, hoping that his agitation doesn't get worse. Eventually I get it open and he dashes out into the hallway, flailing his arms and screaming. Eric comes running out of the nursing station to try to calm him down, but Emile swats him away, going back to his room and closing the door. We can all hear him screaming in there, hitting his head with his hands and kicking the wall.

"Think we should go in?" asks Eric.

"What's going on?" I hear down the hallway, and see Merritt, the new associate director of nursing (ADN) for forensics, come racing down the hallway. "What do we need to do? I'll go talk to him . . ." Merritt likes to talk; sometimes he can overdo it.

"Whoa, hold on," I say. "Let's see what happens."

Merritt joins Eric and me as we watch Emile through the window panel in his door. "I think he might be able to calm himself down," I say.

And so he does. For the first time that anyone can remember, Emile self-soothes. He slaps his head more and more softly, until he is no longer making contact, then flops himself onto the bed and falls asleep. It is a strange way of self-soothing, but he does it nonetheless.

"Baby steps," I tell Eric and Merritt. "Baby steps."

In the nursing station, frazzled Anne is at the computer working on her patient notes for the day. I was sure that the hospital's new electronic medical record system would make it easier for Anne, who struggles to be organized, but she just writes all her notes on scraps of paper and then copies them into the computer at the end of the day. It seems to have doubled her workload and her stress. Her well-worn fanny pack rests on the desk next to her, still filled with numerous bottles of prescription medication. I've seen Anne taking the pills over the previous few months. I have no idea what they are for, but she gets very upset if she can't take them at exactly the right time.

"Hey," I say quickly, acknowledging Anne's presence but trying to avoid a long conversation. I'm angry with her—she basically sits in the nursing station and rarely talks to patients these days—but she gets overwhelmed by criticism and I don't have anything constructive to say. Merritt promised me weeks before that he would talk to Anne about her work performance.

"Oh, hi, Dr. Ford," she mutters, slowly looking up from her collection of paper scraps. "Guess you need something from me?"

"No, Anne, nothing," I say, trying to hide my frustration. "Just wanted to let you know that Emile is in his room. He got upset, started banging his head. I think he's settling down, and Eric's out there watching him."

"Oh, great," she whines. "One more thing I've got to worry about.

You know I'm the only nurse here today? And I did a double last night. What is going on here, anyway? The nursing office thinks that I can just come in at the drop of a hat? Don't they know I have a life?"

I shrug my shoulders and back toward the hallway, focused less on my frustration and more on just wanting to get out of there. Anne keeps talking, even more quickly and irritably. I cannot figure out a way to politely extract myself, so I eventually surrender and pull up a chair.

"Anne, seriously, what's going on?" I ask. She bursts into tears. A few seconds pass before she speaks.

"Oh, Dr. Ford," she sobs, dropping some of her notes on the floor and knocking a few pills off the table. I reach down and pick up the yellow tablets, then deposit them in her shaky, sweaty hand. "I don't know what to do."

In the next half hour, she tells me about being diagnosed with metastatic colon cancer. The staff comes in and out of the nursing station but gives us a wide berth. Anne tells me she is in the midst of chemo, and feels tired and overwhelmed. Her doctor recently told her that there isn't much else he can do for her.

"I mean, look at me," she says. "I look awful. Do you think I don't notice everyone staring at me? I'm a complete mess." It does seem that she hasn't showered in a while and her clothes don't fit quite right.

Kerry, one of the new psychiatrists, walks in at that point. I was told when I hired her she was too nervous—but she has turned out to be one of the most dedicated doctors on the service.

"Hey, what's going on, Elizabeth?" she asks brightly, then sees Anne's tears and stops in her tracks. "Oh, sorry, am I interrupting?"

"No, no, that's OK," Anne says, grabbing a snotty tissue from her fanny pack and wiping her nose. "I was just working on my notes."

"Anne, come talk to me anytime," I whisper and help her collect the scraps of paper filled with vital signs and medication dosages. I stand up and walk into the hallway with Kerry, leaving Anne alone in the nursing station.

22

KEEPING SECRETS

"I didn't do nothin', Doc," Matthew calls out as I approach. He is sitting on the floor in the hallway, his long legs splayed out in front of him and his back against the wall. I am on my way down the hallway to find a different patient.

"Seriously, I'm just mindin' my own business," he says, looking straight at me with giant, unblinking eyes. "Tell them, will you?" Two officers tower above him. Matthew is a tall, skinny twenty-four-year-old who has been sick for a while. His mother tried to care for him for years, but eventually gave up and began locking him out of the house. He wasn't dangerous in the way that would make the papers; he just holed himself up in his room for weeks, eating practically nothing and refusing to shower or change his clothes. His mom thought she could force him to take care of himself if she locked him out. Instead he ended up sleeping in the Port Authority until some traveler alerted the police to a skinny, smelly young man lying on the floor, staring at the ceiling. He was picked up and arrested for trespassing.

"What's going on?" I ask, directing that my first question is to Matthew.

"He's obstructing the hallway; he can't be out here," interrupts Officer Taylor. He not so subtly wedges his six-foot-two body between

Matthew and me, his back almost touching my nose. Taylor is not a regular officer on either of the units, and I've never worked with him before. I later learn that his usual post is watching fifty inmates in a dorm at Rikers Island by himself. He is probably used to having to assert a lot of authority just to feel safe.

"It's count time," Officer Taylor continues. "He's supposed to be in his room. We've got this covered."

My jaw tightens; my fingers start to fidget; and my face turns the color of blood.

"Matthew, how come you're on the floor?" I move out in front of the shadow of Officer Taylor and kneel down in front of Matthew. I see Officer Taylor's fingers twitching—same as mine—out of the corner of my eye.

"Are you OK?" I ask. Matthew nods.

"Yeah, fine. I just don't want to be in my room right now," he says. "I need to get out of my room. I'm just sittin' here."

Matthew isn't going to tell me, but I suspect he is too weak to stand up for any length of time. He was admitted after someone at Rikers Island noticed fifteen food trays full of old chicken patties and cereal boxes piled up in his cell. He tried to resist the transfer to the hospital, but didn't have enough strength. A few days on the medicine service with artificial nutrition and IV fluids pumped into his veins, and he was stable enough to be transferred to the forensic psychiatric service.

It was only a matter of days before he began to refuse meals again. I know about Matthew not so much from his time on the unit but from the daily hospital huddles I attend, where the nursing staff complains that he is not medically stable, makes them nervous, and should be back on medicine. I remind them that one can go weeks without eating, and that Matthew's nutrition will get better when his psychosis improves, but that does little to calm them down.

"What can I do for you?" I gently ask Matthew, eye to eye. Half of me is interested in his answer; the other half just wants to spite Officer Taylor and assert my authority as director.

"Doc, you about finished?" Officer Taylor demands. "Aren't you supposed to be doing something else now? I'm sure you have other patients you need to see."

"Thanks. I don't have anywhere I need to be. If you want, I'll be happy to get Matthew back to his bed. We'll just talk here a bit and I'm sure he'll move along." I look hopefully at Matthew and am relieved to see him nod his head in agreement.

Officer Taylor's jaw is set and his arms are crossed. His eyes are not kind. He takes a few steps back but doesn't give me an inch of breathing room.

"*I'll* make sure he goes back," Officer Taylor smirks.

He is big and surly, but I am a strong woman. I imagine I can probably match him in a fight. Before I knew better, I subdued a man twice my weight when I was a second-year resident on call and he was a patient on the medicine service at the Manhattan VA. He had been threatening the staff for days, insisting that he needed his Klonopin and that he'd hurt someone if he didn't get it. His attending doctor wanted him out of the hospital; I was called to see if he needed a psychiatry admission. We spoke for an hour in one of the quiet rooms off the hallway, and I thought we had come to an agreement about his behavior. I took him back to his room, went to the nursing station to talk to the staff, and put a quick note in his chart. I had already been on call for eighteen hours. Within minutes, I heard yelling in the hallway followed by "Code 2000"—a psychiatric emergency—over the loudspeaker.

"I'm right here," I muttered, and went to investigate.

Three or four hospital police were casually leaning against a far wall. In front of the nursing station stood the patient I had just left, screaming to an obviously scared medicine resident about his Klonopin and the lawsuits he would file. The patient was short and fat, but he had a cane raised high and was about to smack the resident in the head.

I grabbed the patient from behind and pushed the cane out of his hand, simultaneously twisting his arms behind his back and locking them in my version of a wrestling hold. We wobbled around together for a while, him trying to figure out what had just happened and me looking around for someone to help. The patient did a double take, recognized my face, and instantly went limp, slipping through my arms and landing on his ample backside. The cops took over from there.

I don't want Officer Taylor to take over the situation with Matthew. I am the director of the service, and I want to be in charge.

"I need to see Matthew walk," I say to Officer Taylor. "He hasn't eaten in a while, and I need to assess how steady he is on his feet. We should also check his blood pressure."

I nudge the officer out of the way again and put my hands under Matthew's right arm. He uses his left arm to balance against the wall and ease his way up to a standing position. By then, the staff has gathered around, and a few aides come to assist. Officer Taylor doesn't have much choice but to back away as the processional heads down the hallway to Matthew's room. I try to make eye contact with Officer Taylor, but he stares straight past me.

Back in his room, Matthew sits on his bed as if nothing has happened.

"Matthew," I say. "You've got to watch yourself here. This is jail. It's not a regular hospital. During count time, please stay in your room. It's not worth it to get into a fight with the officers. If you need someone, just come to your door and call down the hallway. One of the nurses will help you right away."

I leave Matthew's room and ask the charge nurse to make sure someone keeps an eye on him.

The next morning, I stop in to see Matthew to make sure that he has begun to eat. He doesn't get out of bed. He is awake, but refuses to talk to me. He refuses his vital signs, and growls in an uncharacteristically nasty way to the aide who approaches him for breakfast.

Several hours later, when it is clear I am not going to stop checking on him until he speaks to me, Matthew says, "I didn't do nothin', Doc. I'm fine. Nothing to worry about."

"What do you mean?" I ask, confused. "I didn't hear anything."

"Yeah, good, that's right," he says. "I slept all night. It's all good. Talk to you later."

Matthew rolls over in the bed and faces the window, his back to me. As he shifts, the sheet and his pajama top get bunched together, exposing his right flank. A giant black-and-blue mark spreads from his ribs down to his hip.

"What happened?" I cry, rushing into the room. Matthew brushes me aside.

"Nothin', Doc, go away. I don't want any trouble. I know you're trying to help, but I'm good. Just, please, go away."

"I'm not going away. That's a giant bruise. When did you get that?"

"I don't know. It's no big deal."

"Yes, it is. Any other bruises? How long has that been there? Did you fall? Did someone hit you?" I fire off the questions without giving him much of a chance to answer, but he flinches a little at the last question.

"Someone hit you?" I ask again.

"Naw, it was nothin'. I probably deserved it," he says. "I don't want more trouble, so please just go away. Maybe I'll talk to you later."

"No, Matthew, let's talk now," I plead.

It is too late. Matthew tunes me out.

I walk out of his room utterly bewildered. He doesn't have a room-mate; the nurses said that he was sleeping all night. I check in with the charge nurse and Marie about Matthew's bruise. One of them hustles into his room, takes his vital signs, and returns with the "all clear." He is refusing a physical, and without any signs that he is losing blood or having trouble breathing, it is hard to force him to submit to a more thorough examination.

"I don't know what happened," I mutter to myself on the way back into the hallway. My head is down and my eyes are on the floor as I walk to the gate, trying to put together the pieces of the puzzle. I nearly run right into an officer.

"Oops, sorry," I say, looking up at the uniform in front of me. It's Officer Taylor.

"How's Matthew?" he asks with a sly smile. "He slept OK last night?"

"Yeah," I say warily. "That's what he said. He's got a big bruise on his side, though, and I don't think it was there yesterday."

"A lot of things happened yesterday, Doc. You should be careful. Things can get complicated." He looks me straight in the eyes and then walks away.

I stand there, frozen. *Is he telling me that he hit Matthew? Is he threatening me?*

"You comin' out, honey?" asks the "A" post officer.

"Uh, yeah," I look up. "Thanks."

She lets me off of the unit, and I head immediately to the deputy warden's office. I'm shaking from the interaction with Officer Taylor.

Dep Jones is a few weeks into the job, having been promoted up from assistant deputy warden at one of the on-island jails. She is friendly, yet firm. She got into corrections twenty years before because of the great pension plan, and is planning to retire and go to social work school pretty soon. We've only spoken a few times, but I feel good about our relationship.

I tell her about Matthew and how sick he is, then about the mysterious bruise. I don't tell her that I suspect Officer Taylor—I am certain it will get back to him that I snitched, and I'm scared of what he might do to me. Instead, I ask about video footage from the night before— can I review it to see if there was a fight or something that didn't get reported?

The Dep agrees, calls her secretary, and asks for the footage to be pulled.

"I'll call you when it's ready," she says. "I've got to get legal to review before I can let you see it." DOC legal has to review requests like this to make sure that there is nothing incriminating that they want to investigate internally before releasing it to someone outside of corrections.

"OK, thanks," I reply. "In the meantime, who is Officer Taylor?" I try to sound nonchalant.

"He's usually on 19 South. I think he's doing overtime with you. Any problem with him?"

"We kind of butted heads yesterday about Matthew," I say, and explain the interaction—minus the veiled threat today—assuming that she will understand my side of things.

Dep Jones nods her head as I talk, and then surprises me with her response. "You know, Dr. Ford, I think you and I get along pretty well. But my officers have to keep order here. They are doing their job to keep you and your staff safe. Sometimes you don't know everything about a situation, and maybe there was something going on before you arrived on the unit? What if this patient, Matthew, had hit you? Don't try to be a lone ranger; you know what I mean?"

I want to protest, although I can't come up with a sound argument in the moment. She's right, in some ways, and that stings just a little.

"Yeah, I got you," I humbly reply, also realizing that without anything other than the brief interaction with Officer Taylor I have no proof about the source of Matthew's bruise. "Thanks so much for your time, Dep. You'll let me know when the video comes through?"

"Sure thing," she says and smiles. "Thanks for stopping by."

I show myself out of the Dep's spacious corner office overlooking the East River and walk down a corridor filled with bulletin boards about softball games, overtime, and notifications about recent gang activity.

"Everything OK?" Officer Nelson asks as I head back out the sally port. "You don't look so good."

His honesty perks me up a little bit.

"Gee, thanks a lot," I quip. "Actually, just thinking about a lot of things. This job is complicated," I say, echoing Officer Taylor's words from earlier.

"Yes, ma'am!" he laughs. "That's OK; you can do it. Hang in there."

I thank him with a smile, and trudge back to my office.

Early the next morning in the swimming pool, I try to clear my head by pounding out several miles of continuous and mind-numbing laps. The sensory deprivation in the water and the progressive exhaustion in my shoulders usually overcome whatever anxiety has built up. That morning, however, I just replay the interaction with Matthew and Officer Taylor over and over with every stroke. I leave the pool physically exhausted but with my mind as tangled as it was before.

I don't see Officer Taylor again over the following few days, and Matthew seems to be better; he's drinking Ensure shakes three times a day, and sometimes has an orange juice. I check back with Dep Jones about the video, but "no response yet from legal." My initial rage has simmered a bit, although I spend most of my weekly session with my therapist talking about Officer Taylor. I still think I was right to protect Matthew, but I worry that my ferocious desire to take care of him and all the patients is going to make things worse. Officer Taylor was right that I should be careful. If I'm going to change anything there, I need to choose my actions wisely.

DOC legal apparently never gets back to Dep Jones, and after Matthew stabilizes and moves back to Rikers Island, I stop bugging her about it. I keep my eyes open for Officer Taylor, but he doesn't return, and I don't ask where he went. Matthew's bruise and how it came to be remain a mystery.

23

COMPASSION IS A VERB

Terry stares at me as if I was a blank wall.

"Is there anything I can do to convince you to take your medication? I really don't want to take you to court."

Terry is only my patient for two weeks on 19 West while Keith is away on vacation back on his native West Coast. Now that there are finally enough psychiatrists on the units, I no longer regularly carry a caseload of patients. I miss them.

Terry is so psychotic that he mumbles incoherently, refuses to bathe, and barely leaves his bed. He is charged with murder after someone he assaulted with a knife eight years before—a man he believed was the devil—died several months before. The coroner opined that the old knife attack was a significant contributing factor to the victim's death because Terry had sliced some critical arteries feeding blood to the brain.

Terry's criminal attorney—different from the appointed Mental Hygiene Legal Service attorney next to him now—tried an insanity defense when the assault happened eight years before, but Terry was almost never competent enough to go to court to plead insanity. It's a strange thing about the law. You have to be sane to be found insane.

Terry doesn't ever take medication, unless court-ordered by a judge. I don't know why I think I can convince him otherwise. I talk with him until the DOC arrives to take him off the unit and over to the court-room on the nineteenth floor.

This mental health court is less ornate than the chambers down-town, with their vaulted ceilings, expensive artwork, and mahogany furniture. An elevated bench with a swivel chair for the judge and a cramped witness stand look out over a table shared by both parties and several rows of seats for spectators, family members, and the doctors who are testifying about their patients.

"Please raise your right hand," the bailiff requests of me while I am sitting in the witness stand. "Do you swear to tell the truth, the whole truth, and nothing but the truth?"

"I do," I reply with my right hand in the air.

"Please state your name and position for the court," continues the bailiff.

"Dr. Elizabeth Ford, psychiatrist, nineteenth floor." I speak slowly and clearly so that the aging and testy court reporter won't ask me to repeat myself.

"Thank you," says the bailiff, turning his attention from me to the attorney. "Counsel, your witness."

The hospital attorney sitting across the bench from me stands up, smooths out his rumpled suit, adjusts his tie, and clears his throat. He is a former public defender who shows up every week to represent Bel-levue Hospital in the cases that have been filed by patients. Many of the civilian patients want to get out of the hospital to be with their families and friends; the jail service almost never has patients who want to leave. For them, discharge from the hospital usually means going to Rikers Island. There aren't any family or friends there.

The issues that come to the court from the forensic service are usu-ally about medication. A lot of patients don't want to take their med-ication for reasons that sometimes make total sense—they don't like the side effects or they don't think it will help. The patients who don't want medication because they don't think they are sick, because they think the doctor is poisoning them, or because they are so caught up in an alternate reality that they don't even know what's going on—those are the ones who end up in court.

Being committed to Bellevue, even for those in jail, doesn't deprive someone of the right to make a competent choice about the treatment he receives. Based on a New York State case in 1986 (*Rivers v. Katz*) that relied on precedent from U.S. Supreme Court cases beginning in the late '60s, no psychiatric medication can be forced on a psychiatric-ward patient—even one who is grossly psychotic and dangerous—unless one of three situations exists: the patient consents, there is an emergency, or a judge issues a court order. So, absent the first two, I have no other way to get Terry his medication.

"Dr. Ford, are you familiar with Terry Stanley?" asks the hospital's attorney, standing in front of the witness box where I am sitting.

"Yes," I reply, looking directly at Terry, seated at the table right in front of me.

We're both here in this terrible situation. I am the powerful doctor, talking to the powerful judge, and Terry is the helpless patient. His dirty dreadlocks fall in his face, and there is a ketchup stain on his pajama top. He has bits of paper stuck in his sparse beard. Terry's hands are shackled together behind his back so that when he sits down, he has to lean forward slightly to keep the handcuffs from grinding into his wrists. He looks like a crazy man.

"Dr. Ford, is it your opinion that Mr. Stanley has a mental illness?"

"Yes."

"And have you come to an opinion about his diagnosis?"

"Yes." I was taught in fellowship that when on the witness stand, answer only the question asked.

"Will you please tell the court what that is and how you came to your opinion?"

"Sure. Mr. Stanley has schizophrenia, which is a chronic and severe mental illness that in Mr. Stanley's case presents with hallucinations—

hearing voices—and delusions that he is being targeted and persecuted by a secret governmental agency. His preoccupation with these false beliefs is so consuming for him that he can't take care of basic needs, like personal hygiene."

"Is it your opinion that he needs medication for this schizophrenia?"

"Yes. Mr. Stanley has taken medication in the past, and it has improved his symptoms to the point where he is able to take care of himself. If he does not get antipsychotic medication, Mr. Stanley's clinical state will deteriorate, and his prognosis will get worse."

"Is there any less restrictive alternative?" asks the attorney, using the language from *Rivers v. Katz*.

"No, not that I am aware of."

"Have you explained to him the risks and the benefits of the medication?"

"I tried on a number of occasions, but Mr. Stanley either walks away or starts talking to himself whenever I bring up medication. So I am not sure that he understands the risks and benefits."

"In your opinion, does he have the capacity to make decisions about his mental health treatment?"

"No, not at this time."

"Thank you, Dr. Ford." The hospital attorney sits down and looks at the judge, signaling that he is done with his questions.

"Counsel, your witness," says the judge, turning to Terry's attorney. The judge is one of four who rotate on the bench once a month. He seems to listen to the patients more than the other judges.

"No questions, Your Honor," she says. There is not much she can argue here.

The judge then turns to Terry and asks him if he would like to say anything. Terry is talking to the voices in his head and paying no attention to the proceedings. I watch as the judge grants the order, signs the paperwork, and adjourns the case. The whole thing takes about five minutes.

Two escort officers assist Terry out of his chair and walk him back to 19 West. The ripped hem of his pajama pants drags on the floor. I step off the witness stand and follow him out of the courtroom and past the "Bellevue Hospital Prison Ward" sign. Once I hit the left turn to head into 19 West, I run into a wall of officers.

"Hold up, ma'am," one of them says. He must be new. To everyone else around here I am just "Doc."

I peer through the spaces between their shoulders and see a patient from 19 West being escorted to the elevator, his hands shackled behind his back and his head hung low; I can't make out his face. His orange jumpsuit has "DOC" emblazoned across the back in bold, black letters. He looks like a criminal, just as Terry looked like a crazy man.

"Where's he going?" I ask the officer.

"To court," he replies curtly, referring to the downtown criminal courthouse.

I've never actually seen a patient going to criminal court—they are usually picked up around 6:00 a.m. and don't return until after 10:00 p.m. I'm not sure why this particular patient is going so late, but I'm even more disconcerted by his outfit. That is no way to stand before a judge, much less a jury.

I wait for the patient to enter the DOC elevator with his escorts, and for the crowd of people to disperse. Then I head straight through the 19 West sally port and into the intake area.

"What do the patients wear when they go to court?" I ask Officer Morales, the mild-mannered, beefy intake officer who helped me out with Peter all those years before.

"What do you mean, Doc? Like the jumpsuits?" asks Officer Morales.

"No, what do they wear underneath? Not pajamas, right?" I dearly hope that the patients aren't going to their criminal court hearings dressed in hospital-issue pajamas. How is anyone going to take them seriously?

"Depends," Officer Morales answers. "If they got admitted with their own clothes, they can wear them. If not, we try our best, but usually that's just a T-shirt and some sweatpants."

Morales tells me that I am the first director to ask about court clothing.

"Just trying to learn as much as I can," I tell him. "How can I help these patients if I don't know what they go through?"

Most of the patients who arrive on the forensic service come from Rikers Island, where their clothes are saved for 120 days and then taken to a mysterious room. The clothes don't come with them to Bellevue. The patients who are admitted straight from the street by the cops usually come with their own clothes, no longer wearable after the process of being detained and hauled into the hospital. When these patients get released, they wear whatever spare clothes are lying around in the rusty lockers in intake, or clothes procured by the social workers from the central supply room in the basement of the hospital.

"So they sit in front of the judge in a T-shirt?" I ask, incredulous.

"Or sometimes pajamas," Officer Morales tells me. I think back to a picture in *The New York Times* of a patient accused of a serious crime, standing in front of the judge with dirty stubble on his face, wild hair, and those crappy pajamas. He looks like a crazy man, just like Terry. For a jury, that usually means scary.

"Huh," I mutter. "That totally sucks."

"Hey, if you can help, that would be great," says Officer Morales. "These guys, they deserve to at least go to court with a shave and some clean clothes."

"That's right!" I say, suddenly motivated by Officer Morales's enthusiasm. "I'm going to get them some clothes if I have to go out and buy them myself."

"OK, Doc, whatever you say," he chuckles. "Just ask the Dep."

Dep Collins is the latest hire into the commanding officer position after first Dep Jones, and then her successor, got promotions and moved on. Collins understands that if the patients are treated well, the units will be safer. After a few introductory meetings in which we tried to fig-ure each other out, I told him about Officer Manor. She continued to be posted on the units, provoking countless patients just like Kevin. Kerry had been bringing Officer Manor and her bad behavior to my attention for a while; my file of accumulated complaints about her was growing thick, and my patience with the DOC growing short. The previous two Deps with whom I had spoken about Officer Manor seemed concerned, but took no action.

Within a few days of our discussion—and after whatever investiga-tion Dep Collins conducted—Officer Manor was no longer in the units. I thanked him quietly and didn't ask any questions. Now, I feel certain that he'll approve my clothing drive.

Over the following few months, I call clothing stores and donation centers with no luck.

"No hospital donations," one says.

"We only donate to people who come into the store," says another.

My favorite response is: "Why do criminals need nice clothes?"

Even if I can find an organization willing to donate, finding the right clothes is tricky. You can't just wear anything in jail. Certain col-ors are off limits because of gang affiliations. Bloods wear red, Crips wear blue, Latin Kings wear gold, the Trinitarios wear green. We can't get anything too fancy because patients will fight over it; nothing with buckles or clasps because those can be removed and used as weapons, and nothing that looks like a lawyer's suit because someone could es-cape. Buttons are OK, I figure. They can be swallowed or maybe shaved into tiny points, but they can't kill anyone. I am looking for something very specific—plain collared shirts and khaki or black dress pants. Pref-erably sizes S to XXXL.

One morning, I get a tip from Kerry. She knows of an organization in the garment district that provides clothes for job seekers going on interviews. I leave a message on the automated voicemail. I bet no one checks those messages.

A few days later, I am sitting at my desk sorting through a stack of vacation requests from the doctors and mulling over a staff meeting earlier that morning in which everyone was up in arms because the DOC had tightened up security. The sally port officers are now insisting that we all sign in and pass through the airport-style metal detector before going in the units. One activity therapist raised her hand during the meeting and related that she was asked to remove her bra because the underwire was setting off the magnetometer.

Appalled by that level of intrusion, I called Dep Collins and asked about the need for increased security. He kindly reminded me that signing in and "clearing the mag" are standard procedures that previous Deps had not enforced. Then he told me about an outbreak of cell phones in GRVC, the jail that houses most of the punitive segregation cells. One of those phones was used to take pictures that somehow made it onto the internet. Even I can appreciate the magnitude of that kind of security breach.

"But the bra thing," Dep Collins continued, "that is totally unacceptable. Let me look into it."

About fifteen minutes later, on my way back to my office, I see Dep Collins hanging out at the sally port, monitoring the clearance process. I'm thinking of that now, at my desk, wondering how to relay to my staff that the Dep is trying to take care of them. The health staff quickly and easily blames the DOC for all the frustrations of working on the forensic service, but I am starting to shift my perspective. I know Dep Collins is doing the best he can.

The phone rings. I am grateful for the distraction.

"Hi, this is Steven, calling from Professional Getup. You left a message a few days ago?"

"Oh, yes, that was me! Thank you so much for calling back!"

"I was intrigued by your message," he says. "Normally we don't donate to hospitals, but I was struck by what you said about your patients going to court. What exactly are you looking for?"

I tell him about the patients and their challenges, about how they feel humiliated and degraded standing in front of the judge in torn pajamas or plain white T-shirts, about how they deserve to have a fair trial. Mental illness is not the only thing that defines them, and for many, they do not want to look crazy in court. They want to feel like regular human beings. Steven is silent on the other end, so I just keep going until he interrupts.

"Let me tell you what we have," he finally says, "and you tell me if it will work. We get donations of men's clothes all the time; some of them we can't use because they are too big, haven't been properly dry-cleaned, or don't match. If you can arrange to pick them up, they're yours."

"Really?" I ask.

"Yeah," says Steven. "Really. The whole reason I'm in this business is to get people back on their feet; help them get a chance again. I can't promise this stuff will be what you need, but at least it's a start."

It was more than a start. When I tell the leadership group with which I meet every week—the unit chiefs, Merritt, the ADN, the head nurses, the supervisors in psychology and creative art therapy, and the administrative director—they are all excited. Merritt can still talk too much, but I have come to appreciate his dedication to the patients over all else, so now I bite my tongue whenever I want him to get to the point. He eventually gets there. Merritt is perhaps the most excited of all about this clothes deal.

Carol, the motherly administrator, volunteers to brave Manhattan traffic in a rental van to pick up the clothes. When she returns, the van is overflowing.

"There wasn't enough room in the van!" she exclaims as she rushes into the office suite. "They had so much stuff we couldn't take it all! I brought as much as I could." She motions to the pile of black garbage bags heaped behind her in the hallway. There are so many of them that they are blocking the service elevator. We hurry to distribute the bags to multiple offices before the food service staff or the fire marshal arrive.

"Let's go!" I cry with glee.

"Wait, Dr. Ford, hold on; you need some gloves," says Carol. "There could be all kinds of nasty in there."

I sigh with impatience.

The gloves arrive and my office soon resembles a ransacked laundry room with clothes thrown all over the place into makeshift piles of dark and khaki pants there, designer shirts here, polos and short sleeves in the corner. We enlist the help of one of the temp agency admin staff, a lovely man in his forties who had recently joined us after having moved from Chicago in the hope of leaving behind some personal troubles. He is struggling to make it in New York and desperately misses his three children back home.

"I know I can't," he nervously laughs, "but how bad would it be if I took this?" He holds up an Armani suit that some Wall Street investment banker probably decided was out of season.

The disorderly piles become neat stacks of folded shirts and dress pants. All the ties, belts, shoes, blazers, coats, and jeans—forbidden for a reason for which I was never clear—get dumped in a giant garbage bin and taken down to the central clothing supply room in the basement. The patients at Bellevue who are not in jail can use them.

I call Officer Morales and proudly announce that I am coming over with a gift. I hang up the phone before he can ask any questions, and load stacks of shirts into my arms. That walk from my office down the nineteenth-floor corridor to the intake area, maybe fifty steps at most, rivals the proudest moments of my professional life. *We have done this*, I think to myself. *We made something good happen for these patients.*

When I next see Terry on his way to criminal court, he has his clean-shaven chin held up high and looks dapper in a polo dress shirt and a pair of khaki slacks. Out of his dirty pajamas, having taken his medication for a few weeks, and with a look of confidence I had never seen before, Terry is almost unrecognizable. Even the escorting officers look happier to be walking with a sharply dressed man.

The clothes we get from Professional Getup last about six months, and then we pick up another six months' supply. Officer Morales and his intake officers launder the clothes after each court run and store them in several lockers in the intake area. I keep the extra clothing in my office closets, along with binders full of reports and stats, an old boom box, my white doctor's coat, and a pink suitcase that belongs to Carol. When the hems, collars, and zippers on the court clothes eventually give out, Officer Morales calls me for a new supply from my magic closets. Although he never tells me, I think he is as proud of the clothing mission as I am.

Then one day, there are no more clothes. My calls to Professional Getup go unreturned. When I call Steven's number, there is a new voice on the answering machine. I try Steven's supervisor, and leave a few messages. Months pass, and I hear nothing. I try other clothing donation agencies, but their refusals do not change.

"What's going on with the clothes?" asks Officer Morales one morning when he sees me heading over to 19 West. "We really need some more."

My answer is not hopeful. He sighs in resignation.

"We were doing good, Doc," he says quietly. "We were doing real good."

"I know," I murmur. We are silent together on the phone for a few seconds, just long enough to remember how great it felt to make a difference.

"We'll do it again," I say. "We have to."

On 19 West, a community meeting is happening in the dayroom. The patients are sitting around the bolted tables looking like bored schoolchildren, and Keith, the psychiatrist, is at the front of the room trying to engage them in a discussion about collective pride in the cleanliness of the unit.

One of the patients, Jack, raises his hand. His left arm is wrapped in bandages and gauze from the last time he cut himself.

"The showers are disgusting," he says. "When are those things going to get clean?"

A chorus of "yeahs" rises up from the tables. Ricardo, another patient, raises his hand to speak. "It is not sanitary or helpful to have poor hygiene," he says, "especially in a day and age when we are so advanced and can teleport through time and space while we find the happiness within the great divide . . ."

"Thanks, Ricardo," interrupts Keith, "let's try to stick to the topic. Maintenance is coming to power-wash the showers soon," he assures the patients. "Any other community issues?"

"Yeah, what happened to those nice clothes to go to court? You got any more of that stuff left?" asks Jack. Keith looks around helplessly, spots me leaning against the back wall, and nods in my direction.

"Hi, gentlemen, I'm Dr. Ford." Most of the faces here are familiar to me, but not all. "I'm so happy to hear that you found those clothes helpful. Sadly, our supplier is no longer available, but I'm working to get you some more. In the meantime, we will do our best to make sure that you have T-shirts and sweatpants to replace your pajamas. I know it's not a great solution, but thanks for your patience."

I expect complaints from the patients, which is what typically happens when they are told they have to wait. A comment or two about how this place sucks or how they are treated unfairly. Instead, I look out on the collection of bowed heads and hear nothing. As though they are too afraid or too tired to protest anymore. I feel what I assume is their dejection and hopelessness.

Then Jack speaks: "That's OK, Doc, don't worry about it. We know you are trying."

24

WHEN THE BRIDGES CLOSE

Montreal to New York City is a beautiful fall drive, or so I hear. All I see is a blur of colorful leaves against a backdrop of ringing phones, text messages, and emails that I shouldn't be reading while I'm driving. I am on my way home from a conference on a bright Sunday morning, October 28, 2012, listening to the NPR anchors interrupt programming with alarming weather updates. Hurricane Sandy has already plowed its way through the Caribbean and is heading up the Atlantic with an estimated landfall within the next twenty-four hours.

Along with the other directors—of the CPEP, adult civilian, child and adolescent, and substance-use units—I am also getting regular email updates from the chief about making plans to safely discharge as many patients as possible. The VA hospital down the block from Bellevue, which is slightly more inland from the East River, is evacuating today. Bellevue has never been evacuated in its 276 years of existence.

I place a call to the control room on the nineteenth floor and ask for Dep Collins. He gets on the line quickly.

"Hey, how ya doin'?" he asks in his typical jovial style.

"I'm all right," I casually answer, although I am getting increasingly worried. "What's going on there?"

"We're getting word that there might be serious flooding from Sandy, so we're all here until further orders. We've got an emergency generator on standby that they can bring over from the Island if we need it. One thing, though—I've been going through my records and asking around, but no one can find an evacuation plan. Do you have a copy?"

"Uh, no," I respond. I know how to get patients from one unit to another, and then vertically down in case of a fire, but no idea how to operate a full-scale medical evacuation, especially if the ground floor is flooded. "I'll call the chief and see what she has. What else do you need from me? I'm going to make sure we have enough clinical staff to take care of the patients, and then I'll check back with you in a bit. Sound OK?"

"Sure. Drive safe," he says.

I don't take his advice. I work out a way to prop one of my two cell phones on the steering wheel and type messages with my left hand while my right hand works the stick shift and fiddles with the radio for available weather reports. I toggle between my two work email accounts on one phone, looking for the latest updates, while I make calls on the other one. My husband calls to say there is a run on gasoline and that the subways are shutting down that night.

I finally pull off the road after the third angry honk from a passing motorist and send an email to Dr. Frank, the new-ish director of mental health on Rikers Island. I type: "Due to concerns about safe care in anticipation of the impact of Hurricane Sandy, we cannot accept any more psychiatric referrals to Bellevue. Please hold all transfers until further notice."

I feel a complicated mix of relief and anxiety writing the email. I am glad to stop any new admissions so we can start discharging or stabilizing the patients we already have. There is Jack, the patient with the bandage from the community meeting, who was arrested on a charge of felony assault when he attacked a stranger in the Bronx who he suspected was trying to kill him. He arrived at Bellevue with a mysterious black eye but wouldn't tell us how he got it. Two days before, he sliced open his left forearm with a pen when he became convinced that he was going back to Rikers Island.

Ricardo is also still with us. In addition to the word salad that comes out of his mouth sporadically, he recently had the barber shave half of his head so the intergalactic signals would better reach his brain. The service is close to full capacity, with sixty-one patients who are just as sick as Jack and Ricardo. I don't want more patients coming in, especially if there is any chance we are going to have to evacuate them right back out.

There is another side to this that is just as scary. What will happen if there is no Bellevue? Will men languish—possibly die—without access to a hospital? Does Rikers Island have the ability to take care of really sick people? No other hospital in the city admits these patients.

Just a few months before, an inmate who was labeled as a liar ("malingerer") and a troublemaker, because he couldn't tolerate solitary confinement and insisted on clinic visits so he could get out of his cell, died in an attempt to get moved. His cell had water and sewage on the floor, perhaps his own doing by having intentionally flooded his toilet. A rookie officer gave him a soap ball to clean up the mess. The inmate, likely in another desperate attempt to get out of the box, swallowed some of the soap. Hours later, after officers saw vomit and blood in his window—one of them was reported to have yelled, "Stop faking before I whip your ass!"—the man was dead.

That label, malingerer, is perhaps the most toxic and poorly understood diagnosis in the jail. Once placed, the label effectively gives officers, and sometimes clinical staff, the misguided impression that they can ignore what are frequently genuine cries for help. I am certain there are patients like this now on Rikers Island who are desperate to get help but won't receive it because I am blocking admissions. I feel stuck in a terrible bind.

I finally arrive home mid-afternoon and wrap my arms tight around my kids. They are jumping up and down, waiting to see what treats I've brought back from Montreal. In my haste to leave early after hearing about Sandy, all I have for them are a few toys that I picked up at a Wal-Mart on I-87 in upstate New York. They don't seem to know the difference. All I have for my husband is a tired kiss and a warning that I might have to work a lot in the following few days.

Since I'm facing not only a hurricane, but Halloween, I set to work on the kids' costumes, trying to figure out how to turn my daughter into a mermaid and my son into a cobra while they build forts with the fabric I bought a few weeks before. My mother, who had a busy career herself, made the costumes for her three children each year, and I feel very devoted to maintaining that tradition. It helps me justify the nights when I am not home for dinner.

Our costume prep is frequently interrupted by phone calls and the ping of new emails. Both of my unit chiefs, Gerald and Kerry, are on vacation, and I need to make sure that I have enough psychiatrists able to get into work the next day. When the subways shut down within a few hours, my three doctors who live in Brooklyn won't be able to get to the hospital, so they make plans to bunk in Manhattan. I'm not sure I'll be able to get in later, after hearing news about potential bridge and tunnel closures, but I'm not willing to leave my family tonight. I halfheartedly piece together a mermaid tail while I run through all sorts of disaster fantasies in my head and watch the weather reports on TV. I sleep even worse than usual on Sunday night.

Monday morning eventually arrives and I drive in with very light traffic since everyone except essential employees—doctors, nurses, and cops—are told to stay home. WNYC is broadcasting increasingly ominous updates. Wind and rain are already thrashing Washington and Philadelphia; waves are starting to pound the New Jersey shore.

In spite of the dire forecast, the weather in New York is calm, and I am confident that I have plenty of time to get to the hospital, make sure that we have enough staff, triage the patients who can be discharged, tuck in the patients who can't, and return home again to wait out the storm with my family. Sandy is now projected to hit New York City Monday overnight. I figure that on Tuesday morning we'll be back to business as usual.

At the hospital, everyone is there, as promised. I say a quick hello to Dep Collins as he makes his rounds of the units, and tell him about our plan to discharge the most stable of our patients back to the Island. My office, with its own bathroom and conference table, quickly becomes the command center for the forensic psychiatrists and psychologists. Everyone is in crisis mode and ready to work.

I explain to them the situation the best I can. Rikers Island is a safer flood zone than Bellevue, and can, if needed, fully sustain its own power, electricity, and food supplies. "I don't like the idea of sending anyone back to Rikers prematurely," I say, "but our triage assessment has changed overnight. It's not who is stable enough to tolerate Rikers, but who is so sick that it is safer for them to stay in a flooded hospital than go to a warm, dry jail." I see solemn nods all around.

"So how are we going to divide this up?" I continue. "We need to identify the more stable patients, get their discharge summaries written, coordinate transportation with the DOC, and make sure Dr. Frank and his staff know whom we are sending back. The 4:00 bus is probably the last one the DOC will send back to the Island."

"I'll work on the 19 West list with Keith," offers Manuela, one of the psychologists.

"And I've got 19 North," says another. "We'll let you know who is going as soon as we figure it out."

I thank them all and watch as they troop out of my office and into the units to assess the patients.

Dr. Frank is more understanding than I expected when I get him on the phone and tell him about the patients we have to send back. He is already out at Rikers Island and expects to stay there through the storm.

"I know, you guys are really in trouble," he says, "but we've only got one or two psychiatrists covering all of our SMIs [patients with "serious mental illness"]—that's about 800 patients. All the staff are calling out. What number do you think you'll need to send?"

"Twenty-six."

He pauses.

"I don't know if we can take all of them," he says, "but we'll do our best. They are probably pretty scared over there."

"Thanks," I say. "It should only be for a few days, at the most. I'll make sure we fax over all of the discharge summaries."

The civilian units are transferring their patients to other hospitals on higher ground; I ask the chief about this possibility for the forensic patients, although I correctly anticipate the answer. There are no other hospitals like Bellevue; our patients, the ones in jail, have no other option. So before the bridges and tunnels start shutting down, now scheduled for late afternoon, the stalwart psychologists and psychiatrists frantically type up discharge summaries until their fingers cramp on the keyboard. Dr. Frank and his staff at Rikers Island will need those to know how to treat the patients they are getting.

We have to send back Reynaldo, the same man who kept knocking his head against the intake walls when I was doing moonlighting shifts almost ten years before. He may not do well at Rikers, but he has already started his self-soothing head banging because he is terrified that Bellevue might sink. Also going back are those who are taking advantage of the situation and stealing other patients' belongings, and patients who were going to be discharged that week anyway.

Alan is not going back. He is terrified of Rikers, as is Jack, the man with the slice in his arm. Alan has a developmental history that could break a stone heart. The frequent beatings with a hot iron that he suffered as a kid at the hands of his drug-abusing mother left him with just enough brain function to live independently, but not enough to know how to stay out of jails and hospitals. He figured out as a child that no one cared about him, so the only way he knew to get attention was to create an emergency. The lump of scar tissue on his forehead from repeated self-mutilation is evidence of some of those emergencies.

We also keep Ricardo, with the shaved head; Chen, an Asian patient who speaks no English, who was arrested for criminal possession of a weapon after he disemboweled himself with a kitchen knife in a psychotic suicide attempt, and won't come out of his room without a fight; and one extremely sick and violent twenty-four-year-old NYPD patient named DeAndre. He was arrested a few days before for punching a nurse in the head when he was an inpatient at another hospital.

By 4:00 p.m., we send twenty-six patients to Rikers Island and eight patients back to NYPD custody. The eight going to the police will be arraigned quickly, we are told, and then either released to the community or moved into DOC custody out on the Island.

The news reports say that the bridges are about to close. If I don't make it to the Willis Avenue Bridge across the Harlem River, I am not going to get home tonight. My usual route home over another bridge is already blocked due to a "high wind warning" already in place.

"You should get going; you can be of better use once you are safely home," the chief writes to me in an email. I am grateful for her acknowledgement of the other family I need to tuck in. I reassure her that the forensic service is ready for the storm. Merritt, the ADN, has confirmed that we have enough flashlights, extra water, a few pullout cots, and blankets on hand. He has ordered the nurses and aides who are still there to stay put overnight; they have extra supplies of Haldol and Ativan in case the pharmacy somehow can't supply the unit. Keith has agreed to be the psychiatrist who stays overnight. I already know that Dep Collins and his officers are prepared to stick it out for as long as needed.

The geriatric Ping-Pong table—beloved by the patients for some friendly competition, a bit of exercise, and distraction from the hurricane—makes its way out of the dayroom cage where it's stored. The click-clack of the Ping-Pong ball provides a deeply reassuring sound. The table is becoming more and more fragile, but the patients carefully coax it into its play position.

I make it home just before transportation in and out of the city shuts down.

The evening approaches, and the winds pick up. At 6:30 p.m., the lights flicker and then go out, not to return for eight days. The kids grab the flashlights, excited to go camping in our den, now crowded with sleeping bags and patio furniture. The wind gets intense and loud, but we all feel safe enough to eventually fall asleep. I hear nothing from Keith or Bellevue.

25

WHEN THE LIGHTS GO OUT

"Mom, look outside," my almost seven-year-old son says as he presses his nose against the window early the next morning. Our neighbors across the street have a giant oak through their roof. A few houses away, the road is completely blocked by another fallen tree. Phone lines are down, and cars are crushed under the weight of broken branches. Near the kids' school, a house has been reduced to rubble. Our house is not damaged and the kids and Marc are caught up in the adventure of the aftermath and the excitement of school closings, so I head to the hospital to check on everyone there.

I pull up to the barricade at Willis Avenue and show them my hospital ID. I am quickly allowed across the bridge and go down an empty Second Avenue to the hospital. I pick up some pizzas for the staff near 125th Street, because nothing is open further south. The lights in the city went out the previous night.

There is a huge crowd of vehicles in front of Bellevue—news trucks, ambulances, utility vans, and taxis—along with throngs of onlookers. A few blocks up the street, the NYU Medical Center is dark. I ask one of the news guys what is going on up there.

"NYU flooded," he says. "Huge wall of water crashed into the east side of the building. Everyone was evacuated in the middle of the night, even the preemies in their incubators."

I try to imagine the scene and am thankful that we didn't have to go through that at Bellevue.

I weave through the solemn, murmuring crowd and enter the building. My usual feeling coming in is one of possibility and excitement; now the atmosphere is eerily quiet and oppressive. When the power shut down in the city overnight, the backup generators on the thirteenth floor of the hospital kicked in. They are keeping essential patient care areas in the "H" building illuminated, but every place else is dark. The phones are out.

The long walk down the "F" link is lit only from the sunlight coming in through the dirty windows. At the end of the corridor, the elevators are out of service. Overnight, a massive storm surge, larger than predicted, flooded the basement of Bellevue and rose partway up the elevator shafts. One of the doctors from overnight tells me that you could hear the water swirling and rushing just underneath the ground floor.

Everyone is walking up and down the fire stairwells, dimly lit but vibrant with activity. As I make my way up to the nineteenth floor with five pizza boxes, I pass patients being escorted out to waiting ambulances and a human chain of national guardsmen and hospital staff carrying fuel up thirteen flights from the now flooded basement fuel pump. Although the generator itself is safe from flooding, there is no way other than human power to get the fuel needed for it to function.

I make it up to nineteen, sweaty and out of breath. I had never been in the stairwells between the eighteenth and twenty-first floors before. Ever since 1989, when a homeless psychiatric patient temporarily living in the stairwells of Bellevue killed a pregnant doctor, the doors connecting the psychiatry floors to the rest of the hospital are kept locked and alarmed.

I check in with Keith. He is his usual unflappable self.

"Everything was fine," he reports. "The patients slept through the night; it was pretty quiet. We heard that power was going out about midnight, but all I noticed was a little flicker—maybe it lasted for five minutes—and then the power was back on again. It was really no big deal."

"That's great news—thank you so much. Are you OK? Do you need anything?" I ask.

He shakes his head no, so I send him home to get some sleep.

Next stop is the Dep's office. I pass through the sally port, chat briefly with Officer Nelson, and head down a maze of hallways. *Maybe I'll be able to see the flooded river out the Dep's window.*

He tells me there is still no evacuation plan. The DOC, as an agency that reports to the mayor's office, will not act unless there is an official city-issued Office of Emergency Management (OEM) evacuation order. And Bellevue officials reported earlier that they think the damage in the basement is not severe enough to warrant evacuation.

"Well, at least we're all in this together," I say.

I go to the noon debriefing led by the chief. She has started to run these meetings every three hours so that communication is clear. She wants updates on the transfer status of the patients. It is there that I learn of the plan to move all of the civilian psychiatric patients elsewhere, even the unstable ones. Damage to the basement is much worse than anticipated, the Bellevue officials announced just a few minutes before. It is unlikely that the current state of affairs—the human fuel pump—will last for much longer. The prediction that the hospital will only be closed for a few days has changed to a few weeks.

"We need to get the patients out," says the chief. Ambulances are being arranged by the social work department; discharge summaries are being prepped; and legal papers and prescriptions are being signed by the psychiatrists.

Some hospitals are more than willing to accept these patients, but others need some gentle and not-so-gentle convincing by headquarters at HHC. I listen enviously to these reports. There are no hospitals that are willing, or even equipped, to take my remaining twenty-seven incarcerated psychiatric patients. I start to get scared again, and panic thoughts creep in. My patients deserve to be saved just like everyone else.

"What about the forensic patients?" I ask the chief loudly over the chatter that erupted once everyone had finished their updates. "Where can I send them?"

She looks straight at me, and I know that despite her best efforts, she doesn't have an answer.

"That's not clear yet," she says. "Do you have any leads?"

"Um, no," I stammer. "Not yet."

"Keep trying," she says supportively. "I'll let you know as soon as I hear more."

With no more guidance, I keep checking on the units over the course of the day. The staff and I organize an impromptu community meeting for the patients in the dayroom, to give them as much information as possible and, I hope, alleviate the growing unrest. The update is not very reassuring.

"We don't know how much damage has been done to Bellevue, or whether we are going to evacuate or not," I say very bluntly, "but I do know that we are going to make sure you are safe."

Most of the patients have questions about their family members and whether Brooklyn and Queens are underwater. I am surprised that more of them aren't asking about their own well-being.

Then one patient I don't recognize raises his hand and quietly asks, "What if we're flooded and have to evacuate? We'll get shackled on the way out, and then what if we start drowning down there? Will anyone help us? Will the officers take off the cuffs so we can swim?"

I look around for an officer, hoping that he can easily assure this patient that no one will let him die. No such assurance comes.

The officer shrugs his shoulders and says, "I don't know what will happen."

I quickly chime in.

"I am sure that if it comes to that—and I'm sure it won't—that the DOC will protect you, even if that means uncuffing you."

The patient nods and offers a weak thank you. I don't think he is convinced.

The toilets stop flushing late Tuesday afternoon. Starting on the twenty-first floor, water pressure drops, and it isn't long before there is no running water anywhere on nineteen. The doctors use the bathroom in my office until the stench of urine is too toxic to enter. The toilets in the patient rooms start to fill up and then overflow. Soiled linens are piled up in the hallway. Everyone, staff and patients alike, is dirty and thirsty. I'm worried a fight will break out over a bottle of water. Something needs to change.

On 19 West, Marco, a nurse who is thinking of going to medical school, shows me Jack's arm. The fresh sutures he had just ripped from his arm have left a bloody gash that is now staining our precious clean linens.

"What do you think, Dr. Ford?" he asks.

I look into Jack's eyes. He is scared that we are all going to drown.

"Hey, Jack, how are you doing?" I say. "It's tough here, I know, but it's going to be fine. We aren't going anywhere. We do need to close this wound up again." With phones and pagers unavailable, there isn't an easy way to find a surgeon to sew up his arm. Marco applies direct pressure while I find Gerald. He returned from vacation early and has been managing 19 West.

"Will you go find a surgeon?" I ask with urgency. "I don't care how you do it. Go floor to floor if you have to." I leave Jack with Marco and head back to the Dep's office. His window is now the only place where I can get cell phone reception. There is also a power outlet that seems to be working—an added bonus.

The Dep has been in the hospital for more than forty-eight hours.

He looks exhausted, but he still manages to smile when he sees me. I tell him I have a plan.

"What do you think about moving all of the patients to one unit? We need to conserve water, linens, medicine, and staff. We also need to be able to communicate. The phones and pagers are out, so how will the other units know to help if there's a crisis? Plus," I add, "if we have to evacuate, it will be easier to do from one unit."

The Dep looks out the window for a second and then back at me.

"I was thinking the same thing," he says.

A few of the staff are not enthused about the idea when we gather in my office to discuss the plan.

"It will be too crowded," says one. "The patients are going to fight."

"There won't be enough toilets for everyone," says another.

I listen as patiently as I can, but no one raises an argument strong enough to change my mind. Plus, I think they are mostly just exhausted. Some of the nurses have been there for more than twenty-four hours.

"I know you all may not agree with the plan," I say eventually, "but we are basically now up here alone. We need to consolidate all of our resources in one unit. The sooner we can get it done, the better."

There are a few grumbles, but after Merritt rallies his nurses, the operation goes smoothly. At 10:00 that night, after the final evening medication doses and a quick bedtime snack of granola bars, we empty 19 North for the first time since it opened in 2004. Techs and officers escort the eleven remaining patients on that unit, in various states of mental and physical disarray, over to 19 West, through the dayroom that connects the two units. The officers are gentle and kind, at times more so than the harried nursing staff. They even manage to coax Chen, using hand signals and pressured prompts, out of his room.

Merritt and I stand in the dayroom checking people off the 19 North census to make sure that we have not left a patient behind, tucked in some bedroom corner. The staff stick around for a bit, as if they don't want to leave. All but those providing overnight coverage eventually head back down the 19 flights of stairs and out into the night. When the unit is finally empty around midnight, and the patients have found their new beds and roommates on 19 West, I watch the lights on 19 North go off and head home. Those lights do not get turned on again for three months.

26

A LIGHT IN THE DARK

My kids go back to school on Wednesday, and I return to the hospital, hiking up the stairs carrying cold cuts from a deli on 136th Street. The staff—especially the DOC, many of whom have been there for days—are clamoring for protein after eating whatever chips and pretzels they could find stashed in various offices. Everyone is tired, but somehow still getting along.

At the morning briefing, I again hear about the civilian patient transfers.

I interrupt. "I still don't have a place for the forensic patients. No hospital is willing to take them, and without an order from the OEM, they don't have to."

The OEM evacuation order, by nature of its proclamation of an emergency, allows, and sometimes forces, agencies to act in ways that they might not otherwise be allowed or want to. I list off the hospitals and health systems throughout the city that I have called.

"What about sending them back to Rikers Island?" a well-meaning social worker from the eighteenth floor suggests. At another time, less agitated and sleep-deprived, I might have responded differently. But that day I snap back dismissively, "They are too sick to be there."

I start to think about other options. I try the state forensic hospital, the Kirby Forensic Psychiatric Center, on Ward's Island in the East River, where patients who are also inmates go for treatment to "restore" their competence to stand trial. Kirby already has security measures in place—with officers guarding the front, bars on the windows, and barbed wire around the perimeter—but it's not set up to deliver acute care. If there is a medical emergency, they call 911 like everyone else. Plus, by then Kirby had taken a few of the patients that we discharged to Rikers Island two days earlier—patients who, it turns out, couldn't make it outside of a hospital setting. Kirby tells me they don't have capacity for any more patients.

I make my way back to the Dep's office and find the sweet spot where my cell phone works. I call Luke, who has since left Bellevue and become the medical director of forensic services for the New York State Office of Mental Health. He is responsible for a number of hospitals, including Kirby and Central New York Psychiatric Center (Central for short) in Utica, a five hours' drive northwest from New York City. Central is the psychiatric hospital for the NY State Department of Corrections. Patients go to Central from prison the way patients come to Bellevue from Rikers Island. Luke understands exactly what is happening on nineteen.

"I don't know what to do, Luke," I say. "No one is taking our patients. You know we can't stay up here. We don't have any running water left."

"Jeez," says Luke. "That's bad."

As I look out the window at the now calm East River and hear the Dep's voice on his own phone calls in the background, Luke talks about options. He suggests Central, but tells me it's a long shot.

"Luke, please," I plead, "if there is anything you can do to make that happen, I will owe you forever."

"Let me see what I can do. What number should I use to call you back?"

"You can't call me at the hospital, and my phone doesn't work except in this one spot," I say. I give him my cell phone number anyway, and tell him I'll call him soon just in case.

Within fifteen minutes, while I am still at the Dep's window trying to take care of some other calls, like checking in on Marc and the kids, an incoming number pops up on my screen from an upstate area code. On the other end is the director of Central, offering her hospital as an evacuation site. In the deal for our patients, she includes showers, warm pajamas, hot meals, and beds with clean linens. I am ecstatic. *Thank you, Luke,* I think to myself.

Once I have a tentative plan of escape, I am more than impatient for the OEM to issue the evacuation order. Without it, the DOC won't move my patients anywhere. Unable to reach the chief on her cell phone, I head down the stairs to the ground floor incident command center to see if she's there. I am met with a pair of administrators blocking the door. "You can't come in here unless you are in charge," they say.

"I'm in charge of the forensic division," I try.

"Not good enough."

I wait for about five minutes, hoping they'll eventually give in. Instead, they just get annoyed. I turn around and head back up the stairs. My legs are tired from the climbing, and I have a throbbing headache, but my thoughts are going fast and furiously, if not outright irrationally. *Am I the only person who is trying to save these patients? Does anyone in this city care whether they get out or not?*

Just then, the assistant commissioner of correctional health services for the city's Department of Health and Mental Hygiene comes up behind me on the stairs. I recognize his face from a meeting a while back, but I definitely do not know him well enough to be comfortable wearing the skimpy, sweaty tank top I had stripped down to for the climb to the nineteenth floor. I put my sweatshirt back on.

"What's it like up there?" he asks.

"It's unsustainable," I pant. "If we don't get these guys out soon, there's going to be a riot, and then there's going to be a death. We also have a few on lithium who are getting dehydrated, and a guy just ripped out his sutures because he's so scared."

"That's why I'm here," the assistant commissioner says. "I've been down at the OEM, and they keep going back and forth about whether everything is fine at Bellevue or not. I have to see for myself."

I am shocked. I can't believe anyone is reporting anything remotely like "fine" about Bellevue.

"Don't worry, it obviously isn't fine," he says. He is huffing and puffing along with me as we get to the thirteenth floor. "I think an order from the OEM will be coming shortly."

"This is my stop," he says, telling me that he needs to assess how long the National Guard bucket brigade can last. I get a peek inside the usually sealed pump room and see a ladder leaning against a giant barrel. A guardsman on the top of the ladder is pouring fuel out of a red plastic gasoline tank. He hands the empty tank back down and receives a full one in return.

I say a quick goodbye and keep moving up to nineteen. I report at the 3:00 p.m. briefing about the assistant commissioner's comments, and the chief seems pleased. I get the green light to start planning for an evacuation out to Central, and within an hour, the OEM order comes through.

By then, all the patients have settled into 19 West and are tolerating the dirty and smelly living conditions better than I would have expected. There have been no fights. Everyone is taking care of each other.

The patients gather in the dayroom, and I announce that we are going to evacuate. There is a loud cheer followed by lots of nervous questions about what that means. "Is Bellevue going to be closed forever? Are we in danger? How will my mom know where I am? Can we still go to court? Where are we going?"

"I don't know for sure yet," I answer the last one. It is important for me to keep my word to these patients, so I don't want to commit to Central until it is certain. "However, I promise you that none of us are leaving until all of you do."

Central wants us to send nursing techs with the patients. It's a good idea—continuity of care—but no one volunteers. Merritt, as the nursing director, tells me that he can't force anyone to go because of union guidelines. Central is pretty clear that the staff need to come along with the patients. While I don't hear it out loud, I think the message is something like "If you don't send staff, don't send the patients."

I have until 6:00 Thursday morning, thirteen hours from now, to find four nursing staff to travel to Utica and spend up to a week there. The director of Central, a woman to whom I will forever be indebted, promises lodging and meals for anyone who will volunteer. By 6:00 p.m., Merritt has found two techs willing to go. It looks like twenty-six patients are getting a safe transfer out of here, but there is one remaining patient who doesn't have a place to go.

"He's not ours," says Dep Collins, referring to DeAndre, the NYPD patient. "We'll watch him as long as he's up on nineteen, but if we evacuate, he's not going with us." Because of DeAndre's status as a pre-arraigned detainee, the DOC does not have legal custody over him. The DOC only provides temporary physical custody during hospitalization at Bellevue, according to a city charter agreement from the '60s, because the NYPD does not have its own hospital unit. But DeAndre is technically not supposed to be in jail, and so the DOC will not touch him once he's off 19 West.

"But then what happens to him?" I plead.

The Dep shrugs. Rules are rules. I turn and stomp out of his office—not so much angry with him as I am with this convoluted system that no one seems to fully understand. Limited outgoing phone service is restored once I get back to my own fetid office, and for the first time, I overstep my boundaries as a physician.

I contact the chief of psychiatry at the hospital where DeAndre was arrested and beg him to drop the charges. If he is released, I tell him, DeAndre can join the other lucky civilian patients who are at this moment boarding ambulances to higher ground.

"We are definitely not doing that," he says emphatically. "He put one of our nurses in the hospital. No way."

I call the courts hoping to expedite a trip to the judge so that DeAndre can be arraigned and either released or transferred to DOC custody for the trip to pajamas and hot food. The courts are closed because of the storm.

I call other hospitals in the city, again, and ask if they will please make an exception and take DeAndre. They can legally put him on a regular civilian unit and send him back to the NYPD when he is clinically stable. No takers on that idea either. I report my failure back to the chief, and she assures me that we will find a place for DeAndre.

Somehow, in the midst of all of this bargaining and planning and begging, I make my way home in time to safety-pin my kids' half-finished costumes to their bodies before the sun sets. Without electricity, the neighborhood will be very dark, and the town has set a curfew for Halloween activities. I find old Easter baskets in the garage for the candy, and we make a quick trip around the neighborhood for trick-or-treating.

"No one knows who I am," my son protests. "This costume doesn't look anything like a cobra. I look ridiculous."

"Yeah, so do I," joins my five-year-old daughter. "I can't walk. Plus, mermaids don't have feet, so why do I have shoes?"

After about twenty minutes, my son complains that he is too embarrassed to be walking around, and refuses to continue. My daughter wants more candy, but when I let her go to the next house alone and the homeowner struggles to identify her costume, she comes running back in tears. We abandon the effort, and together sulk home in defeat. I have failed my kids this Halloween.

Later, at dinner, I am still on both of my phones, still trying to find two more volunteers for the trip and locate an evacuation site for DeAndre. Gerald is the designated psychiatrist that night; I have tasked him with making sure that Merritt comes up with the needed nursing staff for the trip to Central and to bug the chief about moving DeAndre.

"We still can't find the staff to go upstate," he tells me over the phone. "No one wants to do it."

"And what about DeAndre?"

"The chief says he can probably go to one of the other Bellevue units."

Close to midnight on Wednesday night, I am hunched over the picnic table in our family room lighted by burning candles. I hang up my cell phone, which I had just charged with the car battery, and sit quietly in the dark. Merritt has generously volunteered to go to Central, and he's convinced one more tech to join the morning departure. Gerald has just confirmed a transfer location for DeAndre on the eighteenth floor.

I check on the kids, curled around each other in their sleeping bags, put my pager and phones on the couch, and lie down next to my sleeping husband on the floor.

I can't sleep. I call Bellevue again to check in.

"It's all under control," Gerald tells me, the frustration in his voice clear. He tries to keep his emotions in check, but I am starting to rattle him. He reminds me of the plans we had discussed earlier, and reports that most of the discharge summaries are done for the transfer.

"Don't worry, get some sleep," he says. "I'll be here in the morning and will get the patients ready for the bus."

"OK, thanks. Good luck." I sign off but am still uneasy. I have been away from the hospital for seven hours, and I have no faith that the plan will run smoothly. I keep hearing that patient's question from the community meeting about whether his life is worth saving. I pull myself off the floor, throw some water on my face, and head back in.

27

GRACE WILL LEAD

I arrive back at Bellevue around 1:00 a.m. on Thursday, November 1. Three hours until the patients need to be woken up, given whatever breakfast the hospital kitchen still has, given medication, and packed up for the 6:00 a.m. departure.

The office suite is dark, except for a light coming from the only workstation with a functioning computer and printer. Gerald is in there, printing out the last of the discharge summaries.

"Hey," I announce before I get to the office. I don't want to startle him. The suite feels eerie in comparison to all of the activity during the day, like a department store at night.

"Oh, hey, what are you doing here?"

"I couldn't sleep, I just needed to get back here. Anything I can do?"

"I think we're all set," he says. "The patients are asleep; the paperwork is all here. DeAndre got moved out to 18S about an hour ago. I was just getting ready to sleep for a few hours before we get the patients up."

"Thanks so much, Gerald. That's awesome. Get some rest. I'll go check on things, and wake you up when we need to get moving." I watch him walk away toward another office that has a cot and a blanket. He looks like he is falling asleep on his feet.

I settle in next to the computer and look at the stack of twenty-six brown envelopes holding medical records, including the discharge summaries Gerald had just printed, and the civil commitment papers proving that each patient is being legally held in the hospital. Each of these envelopes describes a patient who is about to go on a long ride in a DOC school bus, shackled to his seat, with no food and, probably, no water. Earlier, I had tried to get ambulances to take the patients up to Utica, but failed. Dep Collins, nice as he may be, was not accommodating when I asked him to break the rule prohibiting clinical staff on the DOC bus.

"If there's a problem on the bus, they'll just call 911," I recall him saying.

I start to get nervous that some of the patients whose files are in those envelopes won't be able to make the journey safely. *Will Jack be able to hold it together and not hurt himself? Will the patients on lithium get dehydrated and damage their kidneys? What if someone has a panic attack?*

I pick the top envelope off the pile and pull out all the papers, wanting to reassure myself that this patient is medically stable. I am looking for his latest lab values from bloodwork—things like sodium and glucose levels, and kidney and liver function. Also some vital signs and a physical exam. I don't find any of that information in the envelope.

I quickly pull up the patient's medical record on the sputtering computer and breathe a sigh of relief when I see that his lab values are just fine. He had blood drawn the previous week and vital signs just six hours before. I print this information and shove it into the envelope. Central, and any 911-dispatched ambulance that might receive a call on the drive up, will want to know this stuff.

The next patient's envelope is also missing the lab reports and physical exam. I had forgotten to ask Gerald to include them with the discharge summaries, and until then, I hadn't really considered how important they could be in case of an emergency on the bus. So for the following two hours, I review and print out reports to include in each patient's file. A few of the patients have abnormal findings—not urgent, but important—that I make sure are documented in the discharge summaries. If not, I handwrite the findings and recommendations onto the printed summaries in bold letters. I grow closer to each patient in this process, memorizing platelet counts and potassium level. This bus trip is a major risk, and I hope it's the right one.

I take a break mid-review to go to the 3:00 a.m. debriefing on the twentieth floor. The chief is not there, but a few of her deputies and some of the residents are milling around over half-empty boxes of donuts and used coffee cups. The residents, who no longer have any patients in the hospital, are eager to feel useful. One of them, Bernard, who I think is destined to become a forensic psychiatrist, approaches me and asks if he can help on 19. He had heard about the patients still up there. I tell him to meet me on 19 West at 4:30 a.m.

By the time I finish with all of the envelopes, it's time to get ready. I nudge Gerald, bleary-eyed in his scrubs, and head out to the unit. The control room officer opens the sally port gate immediately, and I breeze through. Officer Nelson isn't there. There are no longer patients on 19 South, the intake area, or across the corridor on 19 North. With only 19 West to guard and nowhere to escape, security has loosened up.

When I get on the unit, all of the patients are in the dining room, sitting straight-backed in their orange DOC travel jumpsuits. Merritt has gathered them there for breakfast, it seems, but there isn't much to eat—it's too early in the morning, and the atmosphere is too edgy for anyone to have an appetite. I see Gerald, the nurse Marco, and Jeannie, a forensic psychiatry fellow, talking together in the nursing station. Bernard, the eager third-year resident, is the least experienced with this unit and the population; he looks a little lost standing in the middle of the hallway. The Dep and a few captains and officers are also around. The plan is to begin moving the patients out in daisy chains of six around 5:30 a.m. and walk them, under DOC escort, down 19 flights of stairs and out the back entrance onto the waiting bus. The patients who can tolerate sitting on the bus the longest will go first.

I check in with everyone and talk to Merritt briefly about the plan.

"The patients know where we are going?" I ask. They already know that we are leaving.

"Uh, I don't think so," he says.

I consider this for a moment. We have never been able to tell patients where or when they are leaving the unit. Is this the time to break the rule? It seems cruel and unusual to put them on a bus with an unknown destination in the midst of an evacuation. I feel exhaustion loosening the reins on my self-control. I head into the dining room with the patients to try to relieve the shaking hands and anxious pacing going on in there.

"Good morning, gentlemen," I say in as bright a tone as I can muster. "I know this has been a very tough time for you. We're going to get you out of here as quickly as possible, in groups of six." I explain the game plan, along with the reality of having to walk down all those stairs. "You are going to be headed to a hospital upstate, in Utica, and it's about a five-hour drive. It's long, I know . . ."

"Are you talking about Central New York?!" Alan interrupts. "I ain't goin' there; no way!"

"Can you and I talk about it when we are done here?" I ask, wanting to continue with the game-plan explanation.

"No, no way! I cannot go back there! They beat me up last time!"

I have no idea whether this is true or not, but I know Alan has been to prison multiple times and that he is so provocative when he is scared or anxious that he is frequently the target—and sometimes the instigator—of violence. He storms out of the room and begins pacing rapidly up and down a few feet of hallway, yelling at whoever will listen. I see that Gerald, Jeannie, Merritt, and Marco are immediately at his side, trying to calm him down, so I continue with the group.

"How can I tell my mom where we are going?" asks Jack. "The phones ain't workin' here."

"Why don't you give me her phone number and I'll let her know?" I offer.

"Me, too," another patient chimes in. "Yeah, can you call my sister?" someone else asks. "I need you to call my attorney," I hear from the back of the room. Within minutes, a crowd has formed in front of me and I have a list of phone numbers for all sorts of family members and lawyers. I promise to all of them that I will call.

We get word that the bus has arrived around 5:30 a.m. The first group of patients lines up. Each one gets his ID checked by Merritt first, then by a captain; then each one gets handcuffed to the man in front of him. No ankle shackles or rear cuffing that day—too much of a risk walking down all those stairs. They all shuffle out of the wide-open gates and meet several escort officers who have climbed up from the waiting bus carrying loaded weapons. They disappear back down the stairwell door near the DOC elevator. I am shocked to see the guns, and scared that one will go off. It is another stark reminder that these patients are also prisoners.

Alan begins banging his head against one of the walls when he sees the first group leave the unit. Two techs hold onto him to keep him from further hurting himself.

"We're going to send him out last," I tell Gerald and Bernard. "If he sits in the bus waiting for everyone else, he will smash his head like a pumpkin."

I ask Bernard, who seems to have been very successful calming down some of the other patients, to stick close to Alan and keep him talking and, I hope, distracted from the evacuation.

The next three groups go out without a problem—the last with seven patients, rather than six. Some of them are holding onto their only possessions—a Bible, a stack of legal papers, a pair of eyeglasses—but most are empty-handed. Alan is the only one left.

All of a sudden, Alan breaks free of the hands holding onto him, runs to a support column in the middle of the hallway, and smashes his forehead against the corner. Before he can smash it any further, there are staff all around him, wrestling him to the ground. Blood drips on the floor from his head wound, but he is still conscious. When he sees the blood, he starts to calm down. The rest of us kick into high gear.

"He needs a stretcher," I say to whoever is next to me.

"I don't think we have one on the floor," says one of the officers.

"Can't we just let him rest and then walk him down?" asks another.

"He needs a stretcher!" I say with more force. "You've got to find one." Dep Collins signals to his officers to go see what they can do.

We look at the gash; it needs to be stitched. The surgeon that Gerald had eventually found on the tenth floor for Jack's arm is long gone. There isn't even any water to clean out the jagged wound.

Jeannie offers to go find help. She thinks she might have seen an ER resident doctor on the ground floor the last time she was down there. She runs out of the unit and down the stairs. In the meantime, a backboard has been procured from 19 South, and Alan, now aware of the severity of his injury, agrees to climb aboard. Marco wraps the last scrap of clean linen around Alan's head to stanch the bleeding. Bernard and I are doing serial mental status exams to make sure that Alan's brain function isn't affected.

I have lost track of Gerald, but it seems like only a few minutes go by before he comes over and says that Jeannie has found someone who can stitch up Alan's forehead.

"She says that if we can get Alan downstairs, the resident can get his suture supplies and a nurse and do the procedure in the hallway by the CPEP. Some of the overhead lights are still on there."

We spring into action. Alan gets secured to the backboard, and six big officers, including my friend Officer Morales, grab hold and hoist him up. Gerald, Bernard, and I follow along as the procession makes its way to the stairwell.

"Hold on, put him feet first," I say. I don't want any more blood rushing to his head while we are going down the stairs.

They turn him around and start down. I am at the back, near his head, trying to reassure him that he is going to be completely safe, while inside I am terrified. The angle of the stairs is relatively steep, and you can peer over the banister and see the long drop all the way to the ground floor. Whenever the officers adjust their position—they have the backboard on their shoulders to navigate the turns—Alan wobbles. I have images of that backboard tipping over into the vast chasm, and Alan falling to his death.

"You're doing great," I reassure him. "We're almost there."

At last, we land on the ground floor. And there to greet us, as promised, are the ER doctor, a nurse, and a gurney. Alan is taken off the backboard, moved to the gurney, and stitched up under the glow of the one remaining fluorescent bulb overhead.

I should be relieved, but I am worried that Alan might not make the trip.

"Do you think he can ride in the bus?" I ask Dep Collins, who has now joined us after making sure no patients have been left behind on 19.

"Sure," he says, although I know that I'm not asking the right person.

"Gerald," I say, going over to join him where he is resting on the floor. "Do you think he'll make it? Is his mental status OK? I don't want him losing consciousness on the bus."

Gerald and I go back and forth and then let the ER resident decide. He assures us that Alan will be fine. Alan tells us that he knows the signs of a head injury, and that he'll notify the DOC if anything changes. The Dep promises me that an officer will check on Alan regularly during the bus ride.

So at 7:40 a.m. on Thursday, November 1, 2012, the last psychiatric patients in the hospital, the ones in jail, are evacuated from Bellevue.

28

ON THE ISLAND

I drive home Thursday morning and arrive just in time to see my kids off to school. Then I collapse on the floor and sleep. I wake up some hours later to an email from the director of Central that the patients have arrived in miserable shape—urine-stained jumpsuits, hungry, exhausted—but have now received, as promised, hot showers, warm pajamas, and a huge dinner. When I call to speak to the director herself, she assures me that Alan is fine; they know him well up there, and they will take good care of him.

A few weeks later and I am back on the same road that took me home from Montreal just before the storm, only now I'm headed north up to Central to check out the hospital and see the patients. I still feel responsible for them, even though they are technically under someone else's care.

The director, generous as always, gathers all of the patients in a spacious dayroom with wide windows that look out on the wintry landscape of upstate New York. They are all dressed in warm sweatpants and sweatshirts, some standing and pacing while others slouch in big armchairs. It looks like a college common room. I can't keep myself from grinning as soon as I see Alan standing in the back with his hand in his pockets and a clean bandage over his forehead. He smiles at me, and we exchange knowing glances, although I'm not sure he realizes how afraid I was that he was going to die on the journey up here.

"I am so glad to see you," I gush to the group, feeling as if this were a family reunion. "I'm really just here to see how I can be helpful, to see if there is anything you need. The staff from Bellevue send their best and is eager to know how you are doing."

The patients are quiet at first. I recognize all the patients' faces and know their names by heart, having obsessively checked them off multiple lists to make sure no one was left behind in the evacuation, but I can't easily match all the names with the faces. The only Asian patient there, who must be Chen, sits and stares blankly out the window. I wonder whether he even knows he's in a different hospital.

Jack, whose arm has healed from his self-inflicted stab wound with a pen, speaks first.

"It's good up here, Dr. Ford. They are taking really good care of us."

"Yeah, look at these clothes, man!" says another patient. "Why can't we get this stuff at Bellevue?"

Ricardo, who now has stubble growing over the shaved half of his head, speaks up.

"It's nice up here," he says. "But when can we go back? I got a court date coming up. Am I gonna miss that? They told us Bellevue would only be closed a few weeks."

I almost forget to reply because I am so relieved that Ricardo is talking about his court date and not the intergalactic messages he said he was receiving while at Bellevue. When I do reply, I don't have a good answer.

"Um, I'm not sure what's going to happen with the court hearings," I say, trying to be hopeful and honest. "The courts only opened up a few days ago. I do know that Bellevue is going to be closed for longer than expected."

I describe the damage the hospital sustained—17 million gallons of seawater flooding the 180,000-square-foot basement in roughly an hour, destroying the power supply and backup generators—and that it will likely be months before the hospital reopens. There is a collective groan.

"What about our cases? Are we going to stay in jail longer because of this?" The chorus of protest rises. I hold up my hand to try to quiet everyone down. To my shock, it works.

"We're looking into how to get you down there so your cases don't get delayed. The DOC can do some transport, but we're also going to see about video court. Also, once you don't need to be in a hospital anymore, we can get you back to New York City pretty quickly."

This seems to satisfy most of the group for the time being, and we move on to more routine discussions about how often they see their doctors and why they are prescribed certain medications. I was sometimes frustrated at Bellevue to hear the same complaints every day, but up here, the familiarity is soothing.

At the end of the visit, I offer to take any requests back to the city with me. The patients line up, and as they leave the dayroom one by one, they give me phone numbers and messages for their families and lawyers. Some, like Chen, just nod respectfully and file out the door. Alan, the last to leave, has no phone numbers to give, but he offers his hand and looks me straight in the eye.

"I didn't trust you, Doc, but thank you. I hope I see you again."

"Thank you, Alan, and good luck," I say. "Honestly, I hope I don't see you again, because that will mean you'll be healthy and staying out of jail. If our paths do cross, I'll do my best to keep helping you."

Back in the city, Kirby tries to accommodate all of the patients from Rikers Island who need to be in a hospital. They are quickly overwhelmed and can take only one or two patients per week—many fewer than the usual thirty per week that went to Bellevue. Kerry and several other psychiatrists, a psychologist, and an art therapist all volunteer to go work at Rikers Island. They report back that everyone is trying his or her best, but patients are deteriorating. I go for a visit so I can see for myself.

It's cold and windy in mid-November. My thin coat whips around me as I wait for the Q100 bus on Jackson Avenue in Queens. I'd only been to Rikers Island once before, and that was in a DOC van from Bellevue on a group tour. Standing in the cold, waiting for the bus, reminds me of the many patients who tell me they prefer to be in the hospital because it is easier for their families to visit there than go via the Q100 to the island. When the bus finally arrives, I climb aboard with a few others, all of us avoiding eye contact, as if we all feel a twinge of shame being on the bus bound for jail.

I hop off twenty minutes later on the corner of 19th Street and Hazen Avenue. Unlike most New York City corners, where it can sometimes take a second to orient oneself, it is very clear in which direction I should walk. A giant Correction Department sign looms large on the northwest corner with "Home of New York City's Boldest" emblazoned underneath. Just past the sign is a parking lot, a run-down trailer, and a long causeway that extends out over the water to the island that waits on the other side.

I head to the parking lot, where Dr. Frank is waiting to drive me over the bridge and into the jail. I can only get so far on my own without official clearance—which Dr. Frank has already obtained—or without a specific inmate to visit. Pulling up to the first security checkpoint in Dr. Frank's rundown Chevrolet sedan, we pass another bus stop, this one for staff without cars and for visitors. Standing there are a woman holding a toddler in her arms, likely waiting to go visit the mutual man in their lives—an elderly woman with a cane and a coat thinner than mine, probably going to visit her son—and a young white woman with a tight skirt and leather jacket smoking a cigarette. The young woman leans against a light pole with a sign that says, "The picking up or dropping off of passengers is strictly prohibited."

On the drive, Dr. Frank and I pass two more security checkpoints. He tells me that 40 percent of the jail system—close to 5,000 people—get mental health treatment. Most of it is for symptoms of incarceration, like trouble sleeping, anxiety, and depressed mood, but a fair percentage of the patients, close to 1,000, are seriously mentally ill. Many of them are in AMKC, the largest jail and home to many of the mental health housing units. It's more like a makeshift hospital, Dr. Frank says.

Once inside AMKC, I collect a temporary pass that says "Escort Required" on the front, and sign into an old-school logbook. I take off my watch and my coat and put them through the scanner. Then I walk through the metal detector and hear it ring.

"Back through," says the officer. "Maybe your belt?"

Dr. Frank reassures me that this happens all the time. I take off my belt, send it through, and try again. Another ring.

"Ugh," I say.

"One more time; better try your shoes," I hear. "And walk through slowly and sideways."

"OK," I mutter. It's not the officer's fault, but I'm blaming him anyway.

"It gets easier," says Dr. Frank. "They just don't know you yet."

I try again, and make it through without a ring.

"Yeah," I cry, arms thrown in the air. The officer chuckles, waits for me to get dressed, stamps my hand with black-light ink as though I'm going into a nightclub, and waves us on.

Dr. Frank and I walk down the massive corridor through the middle of AMKC, easily three times the size of the "F" link at Bellevue. Jail personnel—blue-uniformed officers, white-shirted captains, and a few plain-clothed civilians—walk in the middle, heading to various offices, clinics, and housing areas. We pass a group of inmates, clearly marked by their yellow ID tags clipped to their collars, their single-file line in the designated inmate walking areas along the periphery of the corridor, and their occasional stops—to pass through metal detectors that seem to sprout up in random locations. I try to make eye contact and say good morning to as many of them as I can; they clearly aren't used to such a greeting. I get looks of surprise and a few cautious "Morning, ma'ams."

"Do you want to see the best or the worst first?" asks Dr. Frank.

"Worst," I quickly answer.

He takes me further down the hallway to a "T" at the end. There, an officer in the control room checks our IDs, and we make a right to the housing areas called the "quads."

"This is where a lot of the patients with serious mental illness go," he explains. "It's cell housing—so everyone gets his own room—and that helps keep too many fights from breaking out. The dorms are harder, because everyone is right next to each other, and there's no privacy."

We turn into another hallway, also massive, with sets of stairwells and doors lining each side as far as I can see. There are about 1,200 people being held in the units behind those doors. We stop at a heavy steel door with QUAD 18 stenciled in large black letters, and peer through the foggy window at the top. An officer opens the door and ushers us inside, closing the door loudly behind us.

We wait for the officer to open up the heavy steel gate that lets us onto the living area. It's a long, dingy hallway with sixteen cells on each side. Some of the overhead lights are out, so in the late-afternoon sun, the hallway is mostly in shadows. Near the gate is a common area with exposed ducts running along the ceiling that clank and rumble every few minutes. A makeshift office constructed of prefab drywall sits in one corner, but a padlock for which no one seems to have the key prevents anyone from using the room. A few patients are pacing around—no one I recognize just yet.

I feel like I am in a horse stable as we walk the hallway, looking inside each of the cells. The air is fetid, likely from the toilet water leaking under the door of one of the cells. An unused bucket and mop wait nearby.

"This is the worst," Dr. Frank tells me. "Most of the people who need a hospital are living in here. There really isn't any other cell space."

He explains that cells are at a premium because they offer at least the semblance of some privacy in a place where everyone is being watched.

Dr. Frank shows me a few more housing areas a short walk from the quads. We see dormitory spaces with fifty cots laid three feet apart and one officer assigned to watch them all, and much nicer cell housing with twenty individual rooms all opening onto a large common area with bolted picnic tables and a TV. Kerry, the 19 North unit chief working on the Island in the wake of the storm, is in one of these units when we arrive.

"We're worried about Myles over there," she says, pointing to a cell along the wall. "The DOC has kept him locked in for a few days because he smells so bad. He isn't coming out of his room and won't talk to any of us."

I go over to the room and peer in the tiny window, immediately horrified by what I see. A large black man is lying on the floor of his cell, in a T-shirt and underwear, covered in feces. Brown stains cover the walls; there are torn papers and old food containers around him; and the metal bed frame is littered with crumpled clothes and dirty sheets. The smell seeping through the edges of his locked cell door is so powerful that when I get home that night, I can still smell it. Myles is breathing, but otherwise not moving.

"Oh, my God!" I say too loudly. "What is going on here?"

An officer has joined us and explains.

"He won't come out—we open the door to give him his food, but he just won't come out. If we force him, we'll have to get the Probe team involved." He's referring to the DOC equivalent of a SWAT team, which gets suited up in riot gear and responds to violence or security threats in the jail. There is also a Probe team at Bellevue, but over the previous couple of years it has rarely been called; the clinical staff manage most of the crises, and the violence has started to decline.

The officer continues to tell me about the man locked in his cell, on the floor and covered in feces. "Last time we tried to get him out of the cell, he took out one of the officers."

"Does he eat?" I ask. "Does he talk?"

"Yeah. He can talk just fine when he wants to."

"But he's been in here for days?" I ask, incredulous.

It's as if this is not so unusual. I look at Dr. Frank's helpless expression and know in an instant that something needs to be done. If we don't find a replacement hospital for Bellevue, then someone, maybe Myles, is going to die. My brief bubble of peace and relief after the safe evacuation of the nineteenth floor immediately bursts. Even one more day without another hospital unit for these patients is intolerable.

So on December 13, 2014, after a month of whirlwind planning between Bellevue, the DOC, the unions, the state Office of Mental Health, the city's Department of Health and Mental Hygiene, and Kirby, we open up a twenty-five-bed temporary hospital unit on an empty ward on the third floor at Kirby. Myles is one of the first patients admitted. As he arrives onto the unit, Merritt and a couple of officers escort him into the shower and show him to his room near the nursing station. I wait in the psychiatry office, outfitted with a few desks and computers, an operations manual I had finished only late the previous night, and a cot against the window for the doctors who have agreed to work the overnight shifts. I watch Myles as he digs into a tray of food. I know that—despite a frantic month negotiating and coordinating everything from 24/7 doctor and nursing coverage, medications, and housekeeping services to remote access to the Bellevue electronic medical record and a weapons storage area for the DOC—we have done the right thing. I am in the room alone, but I high-five the air anyway.

The next night, all but a few who are assigned to work on the unit at Kirby celebrate at the holiday party, planned months earlier and long before anyone could have predicted a storm like Sandy. I climb up the steps to the top floor of a local bar and find well over a hundred sweaty and smiling people crammed into the space with Top 40 music playing, trays of chicken wings and garlic bread on a table, and a throng of officers and doctors at the bar doing shots. I spot Dep Collins across the floor, leaning against a wall and talking with a few of his deputies. It takes half an hour, but I make my way over to shake his hand. On the way, Officer Morales gives me a bear hug, Eric insists that I dance with him, and Kerry and Gerald convince me to join them for a drink at the bar. Layers of stress, panic, and exhaustion slowly peel away, and by the time I reach Dep Collins, my intended handshake has turned into a warm embrace. In him, I see all the good in the DOC.

"We did it!" I shout over the music as I let him go.

He smiles broadly before averting his gaze.

"What's up?" I ask, a bit tipsy and disinhibited.

"I'm getting promoted," he says. "I'm movin' on."

I lean against the wall with a sigh. As much as I want to be happy for him, the disappointment in my face is obvious.

"I'll miss you," is all I can muster along with my halfhearted congratulations.

"Hey, Dr. Ford, get out here!" yells Carol from the dance floor. She comes over, grabs my arm, and hurtles me into the mass of officers and nursing staff bumping and grinding. For the next few hours, I completely forget about the patients, the storm, and the trauma, and just enjoy the company of my friends.

29

KEEPING PROMISES

I am back at Bellevue, six months after the storm and three months after the hospital is reopened with all the heavy basement equipment, including the pumps, moved to the ground floor. Otherwise, with the exception of Dep Collins, not much has changed. The new Dep, Rivera, seems eager. I ask him during our first meeting if he is on his way toward a promotion in the department; I don't want to invest too much in him if he's going to move on like the rest.

"I don't want Warden," he explains. "I'll just get more work and not much more pay. Won't ever see my kids. I'm good here."

I head out of Rivera's office, the same corner office where I spent hours on the cell phone during the storm, and wander over to 19 West.

The moment I get in the unit, I know something isn't right. There is a big crowd of staff and officers—maybe twenty—blocking the entrance to the north end of the hallway. They are all facing the same direction and engaged in nervous chatter.

I hear someone yell, "Come on, man! You got to put your shirt on or we're gonna have to give you a shot."

At the end of the hallway is a patient I've never seen before. He is about 250 pounds—he could have been a linebacker in high school—and dressed only in his pajama pants. His fists are clenched, and he looks like he is going to charge the whole pile of staff facing off against him. I'd never seen anything like this.

"What's going on?" I ask one of the officers standing near the back of the crowd.

"He just started yelling about something, then ripped off his shirt, and said he'd mess with anyone who came too close."

"How long has this been going on?"

"About twenty minutes."

The rest of the unit is unattended, and patients are milling around the hallway. The worst fights I've seen always happen when the staff is preoccupied with another crisis. Even the officers have all left their posts to watch, hands ready to push the red panic buttons on their walkie-talkies to summon the Probe team. The Crisis Management Team (CMT)—a group of high-level nursing techs trained in the art of preventing violence—is already there, but they don't seem to be having much luck talking the patient down.

"This is insane," I mutter. I hunt around for Merritt and find him at the front of the huddle, conferring with a few techs about what to do.

"Merritt, this can't continue," I whisper. "No one's watching any of the other patients. How come this is taking so long?"

Merritt explains that the patient, Daquane, got upset about some-thing. No one remembers exactly what. A female temp worker was too scared to approach him to find out what was wrong, so she ran to the nursing station, and then one of the nurses called for backup. Within moments, the Bellevue operator came on the loudspeakers in every unit in the hospital, "Crisis Management Team, 19 West; Crisis Manage-ment Team, 19 West." For some reason, I hadn't heard the announce-ment while I was in the Dep's office.

Daquane did hear it, and he knew a group was coming for him. He got angry, ripped off his shirt, and has been in this defensive stance in the middle of the hallway ever since.

"We've been trying to talk to him," Merritt tells me. "Nothing is working. We're trying to figure out how to get him into the quiet room without anyone getting hurt." He shakes his head. "This guy is really big,"

"Yeah, and really scared," I say. "Just look at him."

Daquane is half crying, half yelling, twisting a thick pink scar on his face. His body shakes and jiggles.

"You give me the needle and I'm gonna kill someone, you hear me?" Daquane yells. "Just give me some Tylenol; I'm not takin' nothin' else! No needles!"

"Daquane, man, this isn't going to work. You need other medicine. We're not gonna hurt you, but you need to stop this." The negotiator from the CMT team is trying to stall while Anne draws up an injection of Haldol and Ativan.

The scene becomes more than I can bear. One man in a standoff with a hospital army. Everyone in that army wants to help him—even the officers who are patiently letting the clinical folks try their best—but Daquane doesn't know it.

"Daquane, hi," I call out, waving my hand so he can see me. I'm hoping that a new face might somehow help. I continue to talk as I make my way up to the front of the crowd. I catch a few exasperated looks from the staff—*Why is she starting to talk now? Can't we just get this over with?*—but I ignore them. I care about connecting with only one person right then, and the rest fade out of my mind.

"I'm Dr. Ford, the director of this place. Can I talk to you, and we'll see what we can figure out? I don't want anyone getting hurt, most of all you."

"I ain't gettin' hurt, bitch!" he yells. "I keep asking for Tylenol and no one is listenin' to me. I ain't gettin' no needle!"

"OK. I don't want to give you a needle either," I say. "What do you need Tylenol for?"

"I got shot," he says, pointing to his scar. "Only thing that works for me is Tylenol. Can you get me some of that?" He stops yelling.

"Sure, that's easy." I say. "But I also want to give you some other medicine to calm you down. No needles, just pills. There's a lot going on right now and it would be good if we could just talk about it. Can we please go to a place to talk that's not in the middle of the hallway?"

"Naw, I'm fine right here," he says. "You just want to get me somewhere so you all can stick that needle in me. You're lyin'!" he yells, this time pointing his finger right at me across the twenty yards that still separate us. I am standing at the apex of the crowd, talking to Daquane across the long hallway.

"I'm not lying," I say as quietly as I can so that he can still hear me. "But now I'm kind of scared."

"What, you think I'm gonna hit a lady?" he glowers.

"I don't know."

"That's just cowardly," he says. "I promise you, you ain't got nothin' to worry about. But those other people around you might."

"OK, well, it's scary when you yell like that." I don't give him time to say anything in response. "Tell me about the gunshot—when did you get that?"

He starts to give me a loud summary of having been shot in a gang fight. Everyone around is quiet, holding their breath to see what's going to happen. I inch closer. I think a few of the crowd are coming with me, but I don't turn to look at them. Daquane's posture shifts slightly, and he unclenches his fists.

"Let's go talk out of the hallway," I suggest. "It's more private. We've also got to get this area clear. There are patients who can't get back to their rooms, and I'd like to get all of these other people"—I motion to the staff behind me—"back to their units. No one wants to hurt you. I promise."

Daquane looks like he doesn't believe me. I bet he's been lied to a lot in his life.

"What do you think?" I ask, after he doesn't respond for a few moments. "I'll get you the Tylenol, I promise, and we can talk about all of this other stuff in a quiet room."

He continues to stand there, unsure, and then I get it.

"I'll walk you there, OK? I'll make sure no one puts their hands on you and we'll get somewhere safe. No one's going to touch you."

"You promise?" he asks, sounding more like a child than an angry man.

"I promise."

He looks around a bit to make sure that someone isn't going to get him from behind, and takes a few steps in my direction.

"Do you mind putting your shirt on?" I ask. "We'll get you a clean one as soon as we can."

He nods and reaches down to the floor to retrieve his discarded pajama top. I take a few steps toward him, away from the pack, and reach out my arm to guide him in, careful not to touch him. A few of the staff are muttering and shaking their heads. "She's going to make it worse," they whisper. "She's going to let him get away with it." I want to turn and snap at them, to force them into believing this will work, but I know that won't help, and will probably make it worse for Daquane. My allegiance is to him. I block out the snickering.

"Daquane, no one's going to touch you," I repeat. I say it more loudly this time, to signal to everyone that they better back up and keep their hands to themselves. If this doesn't work, Daquane is going to swing hard.

The staff pulls back and creates a narrow path down the middle of the hallway, so that Daquane and I can pass through. One of the techs tries to put his arm on Daquane's shoulder in support; I shoo him away.

Each of the steps it takes to reach the quiet room is long and tense. Even though Daquane and I are walking, the crowd follows very close behind, fanning out in formation. They are ready to jump in if Daquane decides to deliver an uppercut to my face. I know he won't, though. He made a promise.

We arrive in the seclusion room, tiny and cramped, with a mattress on the floor and padding on all of the walls. It's a room designed to be suicide-proof, with no knobs, loopable hooks, furniture, or sheets.

Daquane isn't suicidal, but it's the only quiet space on the unit.

I hold the door, and Daquane carefully steps in. A few nursing techs and Merritt stay close by; everyone else attends to the rest of the patients on the unit. Merritt tells me about the medication that Keith, Daquane's psychiatrist, has prescribed.

"Do you want to sit down?" I ask. "It will be more comfortable."

"Are you going to close that door on me now, and lock me in?" He is still suspicious.

"No way. I just thought it might be nice for you to sit and relax a bit. I'll stay right here. I'd sit in there with you if I could."

He thinks again about the offer, still unsure about whether he can trust me or not. He eventually lowers himself to the thin mattress and leans against the wall.

"Can I get you the Tylenol?" I ask.

"Yeah, that would be good."

"I also want you to take the other pills, though, OK?"

"What are they?"

"One's Ativan—that's a medicine for anxiety and fear. It helps calm people down. The other one is Haldol—it's kind of like the Risperdal that you are taking already. You know how you got so scared out there in the hallway, before everyone arrived? The Haldol helps with that."

Daquane has calmed down considerably by the time he is sitting on a thin mattress on the ground and out of view of the unit.

"Look, Doc, you seem nice enough," he says. "And thanks for getting me in here. It is definitely better than out there. But I ain't taking no Ativan and whatever that other medicine is."

"What about an extra dose of the Risperdal? You're already taking it anyway. How about that?"

"Why do I even need that medicine? I just want the Tylenol."

"Didn't anyone tell you why you're taking Risperdal?" I ask.

"Yeah, they said it would help me feel better."

"It should do that also, but really it's mostly used when people believe something that isn't true. Like that you're being followed by the CIA, that someone is controlling your brain, or when you hear voices in your head that aren't your own."

"That last one, that sometimes happens to me," Daquane says. "Only when I get mad, though."

"Well, were you mad back there in the hallway?"

"Hell yeah," he says.

"Are you still mad?"

"Not as much, but yeah, I guess."

"So maybe some extra Risperdal will help. Let's forget the Ativan for now."

He is quiet again. I take his silence as consent.

"All right, hold on; I'll get the pills."

I leave a nursing tech to watch Daquane and return with Anne and the pills. Daquane is doubtful and makes me describe each pill in detail, the dose, the color, the name. He eventually takes them, and then opens wide so I can make sure he hasn't cheeked the meds.

"You want to stay in here, away from all the noise out there?" I ask. The crowd is thinning but hasn't yet totally disappeared.

"Can you just stay with me and talk a little longer?"

"Sure," I say. I'm sure there are meetings I'm supposed to attend, but this seems more important.

Keith comes up and joins the conversation a few minutes later. I hadn't seen him in the crowd earlier, but apparently he was talking to Daquane shortly before the hallway standoff occurred. Keith is eager to repair the broken trust with Daquane.

"Hey, look out!" Daquane suddenly yells from the floor.

I quickly turn around and see Terry, the patient who looked like a new man going to court all those months before with his khaki pants and collared shirt, with his arm cocked and ready to punch Keith in the back of the head. Terry is unsteady on his feet and looks almost delirious. I reach out to stop the punch but two techs are already there and do it for me. They walk Terry, who looks like he's in another world, back to his room. Keith seems unfazed, as usual, and stays with Daquane while I call someone to take a look at Terry.

I head toward the nursing station, and then stop, and quickly turn back to Daquane.

"Hey, Daquane, thank you. If it hadn't been for you, he would have gotten punched," I motion to Keith. "We're all really grateful."

"Sure thing, Doc," he smiles. "One good turn deserves another."

30

DIFFICULT GOODBYE

This time around, I know Emile, the patient with the mysterious tics, is coming before he arrives. Dr. Frank called me the day before.

"We don't have any other option," he said. "We've put him in every unit we can find, and he still causes trouble. He just punched an officer yesterday, but he can't go in the box because of his seizures. Everyone wants to kill him. He's got a whole unit to himself now."

"What's that like?" I asked, trying to imagine one patient all by himself.

"Believe me, you don't want to know," he said. He goes on to describe an annex off the medical clinic in one of the jails. Ten individual cells line the walls of the unit and look onto a central monitoring station. The lighting is dungeon-like with sparse bulbs on the ceiling barely illuminating the grimy walls.

There are shadows and dark, dank spaces all around. The heavy doors in each cell have a small pass-through for meal trays and cuffing. "Rec" time—the mandatory outdoor time for every incarcerated person—is spent in one of the four large cages in a cramped patch of outside space just past another heavy door. You can see small patches of sky above the surrounding building walls. There's enough room in each cage for push-ups, jumping jacks, and a lot of pacing on the concrete floor.

"Even there, Emile causes trouble," said Dr. Frank. "He yells at the officers, cuts himself with whatever he can find. He wants attention, I know, but when we had him with other patients, they all began cheering and yelling at him to kill himself. I know Emile is a problem and really tough for you guys also, but he isn't going to make it if we don't get him out."

"We just had him here a few months ago," I said. "The staff is still burned out from that admission. Isn't he supposed to get sentenced soon?"

"Probably," Dr. Frank said, "but we don't know when. You know how long the courts take. All we need is a short admission to give us time to find somewhere else to house him."

"How long do you think you need?"

"Just a few days, I promise."

"I'm going to be hated over here, but send him over," I replied. "He wants to come?"

"Oh yeah. And he wants to see you."

Emile shows up with bruises all over his head and some scratches on his scrawny arms. When the treatment team meets with him, they tell me he is quiet and respectful. He complains about the conditions at Rikers Island and insists that he will be good on the unit if we can keep him for a little while.

"I ain't gonna screw up this time. I know you guys don't want me here."

I try not to get too involved; I don't even see him when he comes in. His new doctor and team are doing a great job. They get over their anger at me for admitting him when he goes two days without hitting anyone. I am thankful that Officer Manor is no longer on the service, and that the current set of officers seems to tolerate Emile with more patience than I would have anticipated. The team decides that it's a good time to try to finally get an EEG. We are all eager to learn what's actually happening inside that brain of his.

On his way down to the neurology service, where he will have to be strapped to electrodes for 48 hours and under constant watch by a DOC officer, Emile sees me in the hallway.

"Hey, Dr. Ford, how you doin'?" he asks. "You coming to see me, right?"

Violating my self-imposed restriction to not get too involved, I accept his invitation. "Sure, Emile, I'll come check on you when you're downstairs."

"Cool, thanks. My grandma's comin' to visit. You should meet her."

"OK, sounds good." I watch him disappear onto the elevator.

The next day, I get a page from the psychiatry consult taking care of Emile while he is on the neurology service.

"Hi, Dr. Ford," she says. "Emile's grandparents are here and he says you promised to come meet them. I told him you might not be able to make it, and he started yelling. Really, really loud."

"Tell him I'm coming," I say. "I'll be down in a few minutes."

Emile is cuffed to the medical bed and has an officer posted outside his room. He has EEG wires tangled all over his head, but he looks relaxed, maybe even happy. An elderly couple stands by his side.

"Good morning," I say as I knock on the open door. "OK to come in?"

"¡Ay, Dios mío!" Emile yells. "Come in, come in." He says something in Spanish to his grandmother, and she immediately turns my way.

"¡Sí, Dios mío! Doctora, le rogamos tanto que le cuide a mi hijito!"

She runs over and gives me a giant hug. I don't know what to do with my arms, so I hug her back. Then we settle in, his grandparents in the two chairs, Emile in his bed, and me leaning against the wall.

"What was Emile like as a little boy?" I ask his abuela.

"He was a good boy," she says. "He always good to his family; he good in school. The other kids, though, they no like him. They, how you say?" she looks at Emile for help.

"Bullies," he says.

"Yes, bullies," she repeats.

"It not his fault he had no mommy. She was a bad lady; we no like her. She gave our baby the drugs," she says, referring to her son, Emile's father. He overdosed on heroin when Emile was very young. Emile's mother was unfit to care for him, so her parents raised Emile as their own. They seem much older than their sixty years.

We chat for a while. His grandmother occasionally dabs at her wet eyes, but she seems remarkably strong. Her husband doesn't speak English and insists on a translation of everything I have to say. They saved up their money for more than a year to make the trek from the Dominican Republic to New York as soon as they found out Emile was in jail again. They are terrified that he might die. Emile rolls his eyes as he interprets for me, but I can tell he is touched by his grandparents' devotion. He is calm, thoughtful, even a little polite.

"*Gracias*," I say as the conversation winds down. "I am so grateful that you are here with Emile. He has had a rough time recently."

"Please, *Doctora*, please, please don't send him back to that jail," implores his grandmother. "He will not survive there. I beg you."

"I know," I say. "I will do my best, but I can't promise. Emile will have to return to Rikers Island eventually. We'll do whatever we can to keep him safe." I turn to Emile.

"But Emile, you have to do whatever you can as well. Whatever control you have over your behavior, now is the time to use it. I can't keep you safe if you curse out the officers and fight with everyone. You'll be stronger than them, I promise, if you can just keep your cool and back away."

"You don't know what it's like, Dr. Ford," he says. "To have all those people screaming at me all the time, to feel like a freak. I gotta protect myself."

I nod, because I know he is right. We can talk about walking away, deep breathing, and positive thoughts, but that won't protect him against a fight with a shank.

Emile returns to the unit a day later, twelve hours short of his forty-eight-hour EEG. The medical staff got tired of his antics, however minor compared to the real damage he could do. They said, he didn't have any seizures and that the waveforms on the EEG readouts were messy and inconclusive.

"They didn't figure it out," I tell Emile in the unit. After the visit from his grandparents, I am now checking on him pretty regularly.

"Figures," he grumbles. "They been tryin' to figure me out for thirty years. Ain't gonna happen."

"Guess that makes you kind of special, huh?" I ask.

"I don't want to be that kind of special," he says, surprising me with his candor. His voice is soft, unlike his usual loud bravado. "I just want to go home."

I become quiet. Emile seems to be at a turning point. He is vulnerable in a way I had never seen before.

"Why am I like this, Doc? Seriously."

"I don't know," I murmur. "I suspect it's a combination of a lot of things, some you may not even remember, or you don't want to remember. I didn't know most of what your grandmother told me. Have you ever talked about your parents with anyone?"

"Naw," he says. "I don't even remember them." His words start to catch in his throat, but within an instant, he is back to the usual Emile.

"That stuff don't matter," he says defiantly. "I ain't talking about this no more. You're just trying to get me out of here and send me back to Rikers. You're just like all the rest!" He pushes his chair back and literally runs out of the room, slamming the door behind him. I see an officer follow him.

"Hey, let me talk to him first," I holler, hoping to avoid a use of force.

"You want him? You can have him," the officer says.

Emile is leaning against the meshed gate that covers his bedroom window, looking out at the view north up the East River.

"Hey," I say from the doorway. "Are you OK?"

He turns and looks at me with fear and shame in his eyes.

"It's no big thing, Doc. Just don't feel like talkin' anymore. I'll catch you tomorrow." He wanders over to the doorway and stands a few feet from me.

"It seems like you were talking about some important stuff back there," I continue. "Maybe we could . . ."

He starts to shake and I stop talking. A few motor tics follow, and then he races out of the room, hitting my arm as he flies by. I grab my bicep to cover the sting and stand there, stunned. Eric is immediately at my side.

"Get into your room, now!" he yells at Emile. "You can't be hitting the doctor like that. Go, now!" Emile scurries into his room. I move on autopilot into the nursing station and sit down.

"I think I just got hit," I say to Eric and Marie, the Haitian nurse. I don't really believe the words as I say them. Had he hit me, or was I just in the way? Tears start to well in my eyes. I had never been hit before. I feel violated and ashamed. More than anything, I feel betrayed by this man to whom I had devoted so much of my care.

I hear a lot of questions. "Are you OK? You sure? You sure you don't want to go to the ER?"

"What should I give him?" Marie asks, referring to injectable medication. "5 and 2?"

"No, I don't think he needs any meds," I answer. I can see into his room across the hall; his head is buried in his hands. He is punishing himself more than I ever could. He looks up and I look away, unable to make eye contact. He springs out of his bed and runs to the nursing-station window, his hands and face pressed against the glass.

"Dr. Ford, I'm sorry, I didn't mean to," he yells, tears streaming down his face. "Please don't hate me; I didn't mean to. Come talk to me, please, please."

I shake my head and mouth "no." He can see I am also crying.

"Please, please . . ." he trails off as Eric helps him back to his room.

"He needs meds!" Marie insists.

"No," I order. "Let him cool down, and we'll see how it goes. I have to get out of the unit. I'll be in my office. Page me if you need anything."

I hold my head up high and walk through the gates to my office. Then I collapse into my chair and continue sobbing.

The next day, Emile is gone. The team decides to discharge him back to Rikers Island. "He is ready," they say. "We were just babysitting him anyway."

Emile never returned to Bellevue. He got sentenced, I hear, and is doing a long prison bid upstate. Years later, I still find myself thinking about Emile sometimes, wondering if he is better, hoping that he is still alive. I wish that my goodbye to him had been different, without the tears, the anger, and the shame.

31

SOMETIMES AMAZING THINGS HAPPEN

I lead a discussion group on Mondays with whichever 19 North patients I can rouse from their beds mid-morning. Since I don't have a caseload of patients anymore, this is my way of staying connected.

"Group time!" I singsong at their doors with a knock that I hope is loud enough to gently disturb their sleep. Mostly I get "no thank yous" and a few "go aways," but I can usually drum up five or six patients. Some are already awake and pacing the hallway; others just want to be in the company of a woman; a few want to come to talk.

After I walk the unit and issue invitations to all the patients, I head to the group room, where I meet Cynthia, the medical student who impressed me so much all those years before; she has since become a forensic psychiatry fellow. Also accompanying us is Officer Sanders, the "D" post officer assigned to watch groups and keep us safe. Officer Sanders is short and squat, with a lazy eye that looks off into the distance. He has been on the unit about a year. Officer Sanders is one of my favorites because he never takes the bait when a patient taunts him or makes a disparaging remark. He has not been involved in a single use of force.

Cynthia is here because part of her training is learning how to run a therapeutic group with psychotic men in jail. She sat quietly in the group the week before, watching as I struggled to keep the patients focused. Cynthia will be running the group today. I will be there for moral support and in case the discussion starts becoming too inflammatory. I think argument and disagreement are good for the therapeutic process, but even I have a limit to what I'll tolerate in that room. There's never been a fight in one of my groups, but I've occasionally had to ask a patient to leave to avoid a brawl. Officer Sanders is very helpful in those situations.

"Hold on, guys," says Officer Sanders, "you got to stand behind the red line. Let Dr. Ford open the door first." There's a line of patients waiting to get in.

Cynthia is already at the door and has opened it, but is stymied by the light situation. The tamper-proof light switch, much like the red button that says "Push to Open" outside the 19 North gates, is a conundrum. Even though a key for the switch exists somewhere, the only way to open it is with something like a credit card. I take the corner of my plastic ID card and insert the corner into the slot on the wall. I wiggle it around as if picking a lock, and after a few seconds, the lights go on. Cynthia takes notes for next time.

The room is on the northeast corner of the unit, overlooking the East River. The expansive views make it seem larger than it is. A broken TV and a still-functioning stereo sit tucked in one corner. There are locked closets along one wall that hold the art, music, and exercise equipment used in some of the other groups.

The closet doors are decorated with patient art depicting scenes like family reunions, broken hearts, and hopeful messages about getting out of jail. Some of the pieces are from a coloring book, while others are originals that, in different circumstances, could be hanging in a gallery.

"One second, Officer Sanders," I say as Cynthia and I quickly shove two oblong tables next to each other and arrange ten plastic chairs around the edges. I do a quick scan, pick up a newspaper and a loose staple from the floor, and then walk over to let the patients in. Most of them are strangers to me, but I recognize at least one. It's Jamel, the patient who was literally trying to get out of his own skin, and who, after he was released, threatened one of the nursing techs when they ran into each other on the street. Seeing his face brings back his whole history in an instant, a history I had tucked into the far recesses of my mind. He looks at me with a big smile as he enters the room.

"Hey, Doc, how ya doin'?"

"Ah, Jamel," I say in response, my smile just as big. He has put on weight and taken a shower; his skin looks perfectly intact. "You look like you're doing better than the last time I saw you."

Jamel laughs. "Oh yeah, except I'm back in here again. But this is the last time, Dr. Ford. I promise." I don't tell him how many times I have heard that one before.

Everyone takes a chair, some patients up close to the table and others pressed against the wall, as far away from the conversation as possible. It's very calm and orderly. A hefty black patient in a do-rag pulls out one of the chairs for me and then waits for Cynthia to sit down before he takes a chair.

Cynthia and I sit at opposite ends so that we can work off each other and try to contain whatever emotions percolate up from the discussion. She begins to speak first.

"Good morning, gentlemen. Welcome to group. This is called 'Dealing With Jail,' and we talk about anything that you'd like to share or think is useful to discuss about surviving in jail with mental illness. Let's go through the rules and some introductions, then we'll get started."

A couple of the patients recite the group rules, not very different from those in community meetings, and then we begin introductions.

"I'm Dr. Jackson, a psychiatrist," says Cynthia.

"Antoine," mumbles the patient next to her.

"Jamel."

"Manny."

"Tyrone. I need to talk about my medication. It ain't workin'."

"OK, Tyrone, we'll talk about that separately when the group is over," says Cynthia, motioning to the next patient.

"Arthur."

"Campbell."

"I'm Dr. Ford, also a psychiatrist," I say. "Sir, what's your name?" I ask the last patient, one of the wallflowers who has his head hung low. I'm not sure he knows I'm talking to him. Arthur reaches out to the patient and taps him on the shoulder.

"Yo, man, what's your name?"

The patient looks up briefly, then looks quickly back down again.

"You don't have to say your name," I add. "But anytime you want to join us at the table, come on over." We don't hear anything out of him for the entire group, although I sometimes see him looking around, as if he's following the conversation.

"So," says Cynthia, "the floor is open. Anyone have anything you'd like to share?"

The quiet feels strange in a unit that is always so noisy.

"It can be about anything," Cynthia prompts, hoping someone will break the awkward silence. Still nothing. A minute slowly ticks by before I open my mouth.

"I know it's hard to talk about stuff in a group like this, especially when you are in jail. Did you know that people with mental illness stay at Rikers Island twice as long, on the same charge, as those without mental illness? Or that they end up in the box more frequently, and stay in the box longer? Or that they get beat up more often? How do you make it through a place like that?"

"You got to man up," says Arthur. "No way to avoid fighting. You got to figure out what's worse—what you can do or what can be done to you. That simple."

"Yeah, that's true," Campbell chimes in. He's young, compared to the others in the group.

"There's other ways," says Antoine quietly from his chair next to Cynthia. "I just stay out of everyone's business and no one bothers me. I been in and out of jail and prison so many times, and that's the only way to get through. Keep your head down and don't make any waves."

"I got to believe you, man," says Jamel. I'm still surprised that he isn't yelling and threatening. He may still be psychotic—hence the admission to the hospital—but he's holding it together well for this group. "I used to fight all the time, about anything. Didn't no one disrespect me. But man, I'm tired from all that fighting. Just keeps getting me back in the box."

Manny, sitting a few chairs away from Jamel, sneezes.

"I'm so sorry," he fumbles softly. "I didn't mean to interrupt. I'm so sorry."

"Hey, man, that ain't no big deal," chuckles Jamel.

"Oh, that's so kind of you," says Manny. "I'm just really sorry to interrupt. Please, continue. I'll be quiet."

Jamel and I are equally puzzled by Manny's comments. I look at Cynthia for help.

"Does anyone else have an experience you'd want to share?"

Tyrone asks about his medication again, and Cynthia deflects. The conversation turns to drugs and alcohol when Tyrone, instead, begins talking about getting arrested for smoking a blunt. Everyone except the wallflower patient has something to say about drugs.

"May I say something minor?" asks Manny during a pause in the discussion.

"Sure," Cynthia nods.

"I don't mean to take up everyone's valuable time in the group; I know I don't deserve it. Thank you so much for letting me speak."

Jamel sighs in frustration. "You fine, man. Just talk."

"Thank you, thank you. It's just that I struggled with alcohol for so long, almost forty years now, and I been sober since getting locked up. I hope so badly that I can stay clean when I get out."

He seems to be a little more comfortable now, and so continues talking. He tells us about being whipped against the wall as a seven-year-old when he didn't do a "good enough" job cleaning up the mess from his father's partying the night before. One morning, Manny drank one of the glasses of leftover orange juice, not realizing that it was mixed with vodka. When his hungover father found out, he whipped Manny until blood seeped through his shirt. But, Manny said, it didn't hurt as much that time because he was tipsy from the alcohol. From then on, he drank as much alcohol as he could get his hands on.

"Thank you all for letting me share," says Manny. "I know I'm not worth your time . . ."

"Manny," says Jamel, leaning forward in his chair so he can see him clearly. "You are worth it, man. You got mad courage. You just hang on and keep going one day at a time. That's all you got to do."

Manny looks like he is about to cry, as though no one except this psychotic patient named Jamel has ever offered him kind words.

Antoine and Tyrone look uncomfortable with this expression of emotion. Campbell nods in agreement.

"Yeah, Manny, you just take it one day at a time. Think about all those days you've survived already."

I glance at Cynthia to see if she is appreciating what is going on in front of us. Her eyes are wide and wet with amazement. We are witnessing a pivotal moment for Manny, perhaps for the group itself. A collective responsibility to care for someone else. No one wants it to end.

32

A STORY WORTH TELLING

"Where is Derrick?" I ask when I pop my head into the nursing station. I wonder why everyone is so quiet. I had just received a page because there was a takedown after Derrick reportedly began a fight with one of the nursing techs.

"In the seclusion room," says Marco, working on 19 North that day instead of 19 West because nursing is short-staffed again.

I hurry across the hallway to the large, padded seclusion room.

I see Derrick, covered in bloody sheets, lying on a makeshift bed in a fetal position. His ill-fitting and blood-stained pajama bottoms have slipped below his hips, but he doesn't seem to notice. It looks like he is asleep, but his eyes are so swollen and bloody that I can't tell. Blood has crusted around his face, particularly in his scruffy beard, and is turning as black as his skin. He looks like a bloody baby.

I run back to the nursing station to get a pair of gloves, but all the boxes are empty.

"Hey, we need more gloves," I yell. A few minutes later, a box of size medium appears.

"Give me a break," I mutter, jamming my fingers into the purple latex. I have very long fingers and always use L or XL.

"How long has he been like this?" I ask the tech standing guard just outside the room. He is new.

"I don't know," he says in a thick East African accent, stumbling over his words. "I just took over. Let me go check." He begins to head back across the hallway.

"No," I stop him. "That's OK. Can you just call someone from the nursing station to come over?"

I wonder why nobody has bothered to get Derrick out of the bloody sheets or clean him up. *Has he done something so terrible that no one is willing to help him?*

"Derrick," I coo, approaching him slowly.

He is a big man, well over 6 feet and close to 250 pounds.

"Derrick," I say again, this time a little louder. "I'm Dr. Ford. I need to look you over and see where you're hurt. Can you hear me?"

He nods weakly. In addition to whatever had happened earlier, Derrick had also received an injection of Haldol and Ativan, so he is nearly asleep.

"OK, good. I'm probably going to need your help a little bit." I turn to the tech to ask for help, but he looks too scared to do anything.

"Let's just roll you on your back. Gently. Does that hurt?" Derrick slowly positions himself on his back as I help to move his hips around.

I start at his feet and work my way up, checking for bruises, any movement restrictions, any pain. I gently prod his abdomen and his lower back, careful about the risk of internal bleeding. He winces when I push on the left side, near the spleen.

"Does that hurt?" I ask. I can't make out his response.

Just then, Kerry walks in. She saw Derrick earlier in the morning and has already paged the plastic surgeon to take a look at his eye. She has the glazed look in her own eyes that I have come to know as her response to panic. She temporarily seals over to not have to feel the horror that she is experiencing.

"Can you order an abdominal CT for him?" I ask. "He's tender on the left side." It is a long shot that he has any internal bleeding—his vital signs are stable—but I am not going to let anything get missed. Kerry says she will add it to the face CT she already ordered.

I open Derrick's pajama top and see some bruising around his ribs. His skin is clammy.

Then I look at his face in more detail. He has dried blood everywhere, although it looks like the source is largely a cut to his lip and one above his eyebrow. The eyebrow laceration is pretty deep, and the skin around his eyes is mottled and bruised. Both eyelids are swollen shut, but Derrick lets me peel them back, or at least doesn't swat me away.

The pupils look OK, a good sign. I have seen many head injuries over the years, but have never, luckily, seen a blown pupil. That happens when your brain starts swelling through the hole in the bottom of your skull and the nerves in the brainstem that control pupillary reflexes get compressed. Without quick neurosurgical intervention, it usually means imminent death.

From the look of Derrick's injuries, he has been beaten up. No takedown in a hospital should involve multiple blows to the head. The staff, ordinarily extremely efficient with emergencies and trauma care, seem particularly wary and passive this morning. Something has happened, and no one is talking about it.

Derrick whispers a few words as I examine his face.

"What did you say?" I lean in closer, my ear inches from his bloody lips.

"I'm sorry," he quietly pleads. "It wasn't my fault." Tears are leaking through his swollen lids.

I am speechless, struggling to keep my cool in the face of what I am convinced is foul play. This can't have just been a takedown. Soon I will start an investigation and all the eyewitnesses will at first say they saw nothing improper. Then the accusations will start to fly. For now, though, I kneel next to Derrick, hold his hand, and instinctively begin rubbing my thumb back and forth against his palm, the way my children love for me to do when I am putting them to sleep.

Eventually, we—the Chief becomes involved—learn what happened. I am devastated, but not altogether surprised, given the incredible pressure of working in these units. Just as, at the time, I kept my findings as confidential as possible to protect the safety of my patients and the staff, so must I now do the same. A story without an ending is unsatisfying and incomplete. Yet, like the stories of so many of my patients whose endings I do not know—those of Emile, Jamel, Alan, Eaton, and many more—it is still a story worth telling.

33

HIGHER POWER

Javon faces me on the other side of a ticket-booth-type Plexiglas partition in a largely unused interview room on 19 West. The more spacious room with the table, the one where Simmons threw a chair at me while I was pregnant, is taken. There are speaker holes in the partition here, but two of them are clogged with spitballs, and I can barely hear what Javon is saying. I scoot forward on the edge of my chair, my legs tangled up under me, and bring my face as close to the partition as possible without actually touching it.

"Hi, Javon," I begin. "I'm sorry about the room setup here. It's all we have for now. Hopefully it won't be too bad."

I change my tone for the next question—softer, more soothing. "How was your night?"

I am checking in because I know he was found guilty of murder the day before and may be facing a life sentence.

Javon looks at the ground for a moment, collects his thoughts, and surprises me with his question back.

"Do you believe in God?" he asks.

My religious life flashes past in a few milliseconds as I try to formulate my answer. Sunday school as a kid making paper arks and listening to stories about Jesus, skipping out on actual church with my brother and father to get Dunkin' Donuts, attending mass on occasion with my Catholic best friend and being puzzled by all of the ritual. Then, while living in Egypt as a teenager and visiting the Church of the Holy Sepulchre, the Dome of the Rock, and the Wailing Wall in Jerusalem, feeling for the first time in my life the presence of a higher power.

"I don't really know, Javon. I'm still trying to figure it out." That is the most honest answer I can give.

"Well, let me help you," he says. "My life changed yesterday, but not in the way you think. I finally got what I been waiting for. I been sitting in this shithole jail for two years with no one tellin' me nothin', and then yesterday I finally got an answer. Do I like the answer? Naw, that would be downright stupid. But I sure do like knowin'. And God gave me that. He gave me faith in him, that he's got my back no matter what. He knew that I needed an answer, and he gave it to me. I slept like a baby last night, Doc."

I am speechless.

"Come on, Doc, it's not that big a deal. Don't worry about it."

My eyes are wet, with tears not of sorrow, but relief. I am relieved that he will survive, that I won't be up nights worrying whether he will be another Franklin. Javon's faith in a higher power will help him make it through the rest of his imprisoned life with restful nights. My doctoring skills don't come close to his belief in God.

34

PING-PONG THERAPY

The Ping-Pong table has been broken, repaired, and rebroken more times than anyone can count. Unlike most of the other things that frequently break in the unit—windows, toilets, noses—the repeated destruction of the Ping-Pong table has nothing to do with the patients. The table is just too old to tolerate its daily folding and unfolding.

One day, the table's tarnished hinges give out. The head of activity therapy, Carl, brings in a parade of engineers, facility managers, and anyone with a racket-sport background in an attempt to bring the table back to life. The prognosis is dire. Carl and a few colleagues roll the unresponsive table up to the equipment graveyard in a storage closet on the twenty-first floor.

The following few months are grim. Every community meeting, a patient asks about the Ping-Pong table. "When is it coming back? What is taking so long? Can't we just use the broken one again?"

Although I have no proof, I speculate that our rates of violence are directly linked to the presence of that table. It has an uncanny knack of calming everyone down. Who can resist the playful pull of that tiny white ball skimming across a smooth green surface? The hospital refuses to pay for another table, citing financial hardship and insisting that the table is a "nonessential" expense. The DOC says it's not responsible for this extravagant kind of purchase.

Then, one day, Carl bursts into the conference room, unable to contain his excitement. Through an anonymous tip received from an unnamed friend who allegedly has ties to the National Ping Pong Association, Carl receives a donation of a competition-grade Ping-Pong table. Within a few days, he is going to pick it up from the back entrance of a nondescript warehouse somewhere in midtown Manhattan. I let out a joyous scream and throw my hands in the air in delight. We are saved!

My joy is short-lived. The Dep won't allow the net on the unit.

"Can't take the risk of a hang-up or a fight," he tells me. "Find me a net that works, and you're in business."

I bring the challenge back to Merritt, the unit chiefs, Carl, and the director of psychology.

"How about we draw a net on a long piece of cardboard?" Carl offers. "How much damage can you do with compressed paper?"

"What if they just played without a net?" asks the head of psychology.

"How about we substitute a medication discussion group for Ping-Pong?" quips Merritt.

"What if we just use the net we have and hope the Dep doesn't notice?" suggests Kerry.

I leave the meeting prepared to make another pitch to Dep Rivera about the urgent need for us to get the table into action. He is waiting at my office door.

"Can we talk about the . . ."

"I think I have the answer for the Ping-Pong table," he interrupts. "I just went to look at it again."

"Oh, that's awesome. What is your idea?"

"Noodles."

"What? A net made out of noodles?" I have no idea what he is talking about.

"No, no. You know those Styrofoam noodles that kids play with in the pool? The long ones with the holes in the middle?"

"Yeah." I have no idea how this relates to Ping-Pong.

"If you cut one of those and hot glue the net to the ends, you've got yourself a net!"

"I don't understand anything you've just told me."

He explains again, but I still can't grasp the concept. Every time he says "noodle," I start to giggle.

"You know what?" I finally say, pulling myself together. "I don't know how you plan to build this net, but the fact that you're so into it is pretty cool. Why don't we try it?"

We set a time for the following week to meet at the new table. A few days later, I find an orange noodle on my desk. I call Carl and Mary Beth—the new and very crafty administrator for the forensic psychiatry service. She shows up with her hot glue gun. Carl has a range of net choices, and I have an X-Acto knife in my blazer pocket and the orange noodle over my shoulder. Dep Rivera appears with his white sleeves rolled to the elbow and a set of tools in hand.

The construction project begins. The Dep starts to cut the noodle into 18-inch pieces, explaining that they are going to be the net posts. He wedges them vertically into the center gap of the partially folded table, one on each side, straightens out the table, and voilà! Orange foam posts. The only safety hazard I can imagine is the risk that a patient might try to eat the polyethylene foam. Those noodles at the pool always have bite marks in them.

Mary Beth and I loop the ends of one of the nets over the noodle posts, and the Dep refines the posts slightly with small cuts from the X-Acto knife. We practice inserting the noodle net a few times so that Carl can demonstrate to his staff and step back to admire our handiwork. *Welcome to your new life, Ping-Pong table!*

Although the patients look at us—the Dep, Mary Beth, Carl, and me—like we have lost our minds when we proudly roll the table into the dayroom, it doesn't take long before there is a waiting list for matches. The table gets used for over an hour straight, and at the end of the frenzy, the noodle net is in pieces, orange foam littered all over the floor. I am crestfallen, but Carl quickly creates a cardboard net—his original idea—and the games continue. I leave the patients happily slapping the Ping-Pong ball back and forth, unaware of the group effort that went into its creation. Back at my office, I take out the small piece of orange foam stuffed in my pocket and gently place it on a shelf next to an hourglass I received when I graduated from psychiatric residency and photographs of my children.

35

A BRIGHTER DAY

Today is a performance community meeting, a talent show of sorts. The green plastic chairs are arranged in a haphazard circle in the dayroom. The leader of the meeting, a plucky young drama therapist named Cordell, and the performers, who have rehearsed with her earlier in the day, are in the room, talking quietly in a corner.

Lee, a patient, sits in one of the giant green chairs. He is older than me, although we both have graying hair around the temples. I sit down next to him and offer a smile. He wears his flimsy hospital pajamas and is hunched over, staring at the floor. He is clutching two pieces of paper—one a memo from the DOC's phone center bearing the handwritten message "Your mother called and would like you to call her back," and the other a copy of the lyrics to "We Are the World." We sit side by side for several minutes. At least one of us is thinking of the many states of being that separate us—patient and doctor, man and woman, black and white, mentally ill and healthy, incarcerated and free.

Patients drift in slowly at first, then more quickly.

"Welcome to the community meeting," Cordell begins in a chipper voice. She's smiling broadly, though there is a tension in the room.

Since life on 19 West depends largely on the patients, our major goal is to inspire them to get along, with each other, and with us. And since we can't reward their good behavior with material goods like food, money, or magazines—DOC orders—we search for intangible rewards like pride, respect, and leadership. Patients who behave well get certificates of merit, they get to colead community meetings, and, for our most popular offering, they get to perform.

Patients who follow their treatment plans and stay out of fights are invited to rap, sing, act, show their artwork, or recite poetry in front of an audience of their peers, the clinical staff, and occasionally, the DOC officers. The staff were skeptical about the value of a talent show as a reward—"It don't taste as good as McDonald's"—but they were at least willing to try. Now they are totally convinced.

Cordell, who inspired and encouraged the performance community meetings, gets things going. First up are three poets: a young black man whom I recognize, a young white man with ill-fitting glasses and tousled red hair, and an elderly Hispanic man who hoists himself up from his wheelchair. They each recite several verses from a poem they had written together over the course of the week. Solemn yet thankful, their poem chronicles their lives and stories of poverty, abuse, and incarceration. When they are done, they receive a polite round of applause.

"Now we'd like everyone to stand up," Cordell announces. The staff are uneasy but oblige her request; a few of the patients decide to stay in their seats.

"Please look at the lyrics we left on your chairs," Cordell directs, referring to "We Are the World," a copy of which Lee still has. Since there are not enough sheets to go around, we are directed to share with our neighbor. My only neighbor is Lee. He hands me the lyrics sheet, then looks away.

"Do you want to share?" I ask.

"No," he mutters, shaking his head and turning his gaze to the floor.

"The performers have requested that we all sing together," Cordell continues.

I have a deep-rooted fear of singing, thanks to a school chorus audition in the sixth grade. I was laughed off the stage, never to sing publicly again. When I'm in the car with my children and I start singing to the radio, they hold their hands over their ears and beg me to stop.

The music track comes on. I start singing softly, tentatively. I try to follow along with Lionel Richie, and take some inexplicable comfort from Lee's quiet presence next to me.

At the end of the first chorus, I look around the room. It is clear that the song is affecting the patients. Lee has started to sing, a hint of a smile on his face. Another patient, a man with gauze-covered cut marks on his arms, flanked by a tech doing suicide watch, has tears trickling down his grinning face. By the third chorus—we've just finished the line "Let's realize that a change can only come when we stand together as one"—the nervous tension that had filled the room in the beginning starts to dissipate. Patients and staff are clapping their hands; the voices are getting louder; and I am singing at the top of my lungs. Even the officer in the corner is singing along.

I am tempted to pump my fist in the air and shout. A patient yells, "Come on, everyone, one more time!" The three patient-performers who had earned the privilege of directing the group-sing are beaming. And to my left there is Lee, singing and peaceful.

"There's a choice we're making. We're saving our own lives."

36

BEYOND BELLEVUE

My thoughts are heavy as I begin my commute home, walking up First Avenue to the train station, past the ambulance lane on 28th Street and the renovated Administration of Children and Family Services building. It is a reception center and intake facility for abused, neglected, and abandoned children. I am afraid that if I see a child being taken inside, I will swirl into a panic of implications, so I keep my head down as I go by.

I look up as I approach 30th Street and the Bellevue Men's Shelter, the central triage point for the homeless of New York City. It was formerly the Bellevue Psychiatric Hospital; the ornate wrought-iron gates along First Avenue hint at long-lost architectural grandeur. Now it is covered in weeds, with discarded cigarette butts and pieces of broken marble pillars leaning haphazardly against the gates and the building walls. In the late-afternoon shadows, the courtyard gets dark and eerie.

I think of the offer I had received earlier that day as I stand on the corner and wait to cross the street. The assistant commissioner for correctional health services, the same man who had trudged up the stairs with me in the aftermath of Sandy, had called to say that he wants me to help reform the mental health care at Rikers Island. He tells me the city's new mayor has his eye on the jail; there is a new commissioner of health, and, starting the following week, there will be a new commissioner for the DOC. I think about Myles, the man we discovered lying in his own feces in a locked cell after the storm.

I think about a 39-year-old man with schizophrenia and diabetes who died after being locked in his cell for days. On day seven, he was discovered unresponsive with a ligature tied around his swollen and infected genitalia. And just two months ago, a fifty-six-year-old man taking heat-sensitive antipsychotic medication and arrested for trespassing, was found dead in his overheated cell. Even though I am not looking for a new job, the lure of this kind of challenge is compelling. My patients at Bellevue almost always start and end their jail journeys on Rikers Island. *Maybe I should think about moving to the source?*

I hear my name called from across the street and snap out of my thoughts. It sounds distant and muffled. I look around but just see the usual cadre of homeless men enjoying the early spring air and a smoke before darkness settles and they have to go back inside.

"Dr. Ford, yo, wait a second!" I hear again.

This time the words are much clearer and aren't from across the street. They are right next to me.

"Oh my God, Jamel, how are you?" I stammer. He is dressed in a red bomber jacket over a checkered button-down on top of a T-shirt. His jeans are slung low, and he has on fresh Timberlands. If it hadn't been for his face, fuller than I remembered from his last hospitalization, I would never have recognized him. With his backpack over one shoulder, he looks a bit like a college kid.

"I'm hangin' in there," he says. "Trying to figure everything out. I just had a baby girl not too long ago." A big grin appears on his face.

"Oh, that's wonderful!" I say. "Congratulations!" I am struck by how little he resembles a psychiatric patient.

"You look terrific. Are you working?"

"Sort of," he says. "Just some odd jobs here and there. I'm taking my medication, though," he announces with great satisfaction. "You remember that clozapine stuff you started?"

I slowly nod, also remembering why I stopped it.

"They tried it again—I guess you can do that after a while—and it's working. I ain't sick at all; my blood counts look good; and I ain't been arrested in six months. What do you think of that, Doc?"

I want more than anything to give him a big hug.

"Amazing!" I cry. "You feel OK on it? Do you like your doctor?"

"Yeah, yeah, that's all good. I even told my mom; I said, 'Dr. Ford would be proud of me.'"

I gaze at him, still shocked at how well he has done. I don't want the moment to end.

"I've got to get home," I tell him anyway, aware that I am still his former doctor and he is my former patient.

"Yeah, me too," he says. "Maybe I'll see you around?"

"I hope so." We shake hands and smile. I head north up First Avenue, crossing 30th Street and then stopping at the light. I look back and see him standing there, waving goodbye.

That night, without telling anyone and only barely realizing it myself, I decide that I am going to leave Bellevue. The tug of what's out there at Rikers Island, even if it's only desperation and chaos, is too strong. If Bellevue can help a man like Jamel, with incredible doctors who love what they do and officers who have accepted the safety of respect and kindness, it doesn't need me anymore.

I wanted a sign to help me make this decision, and Jamel just gave me one.

EPILOGUE

I had been to Rikers Island before, but it feels like I am seeing things for the first time. I am no longer a tourist there; I am about to become one of the natives.

In front of me stretches an elegant, two-lane causeway that gently arches up and over the western fingers of the Long Island Sound. Seagulls soar near the railings of the bridge. If the temperature had been a few degrees warmer, the water a little bit more blue, and the drivers a few years older, I could have been traveling over San Carlos Bay in the Gulf of Mexico to the beautiful sandy beaches of Florida's Sanibel Island. But there aren't any beaches where I am going.

To the right, the crisscrossing runways of LaGuardia airport welcome and then disperse hundreds of airplanes each day. To the left, spewing either smoke or flames into the New York air, is a water treatment plant. But straight ahead, accessible only by this sliver of a road, is the island that is a temporary home for more than 100,000 people a year.

Three giant buildings rise above the other low-slung structures, two twins at the eastern edge of the island and a third on the western edge, overlooking the Manhattan skyline. This western facility houses mostly individuals who are locked in solitary confinement, yet it has the best riverfront views available. Perhaps this is intentional; the majestic scene might soothe the restless minds of the people who live there. At night, when the twinkly lights start to illuminate the East River, you can hear the residents howling, as if the city were the moon.

The island is heavily guarded, although with the right credentials—mine arrived the day before—it takes about ten seconds to show my IDs, say good morning, and drive right through the security checkpoint. I navigate over the moveable speed bumps arranged in uneven zigzags, a new configuration every day. I underestimate the impact of these bumps and nearly take out one of my axles.

A white school bus passes me and then stops to drop off and pick up passengers. That must be the 24-hour shuttle bus, always available to transport carless visitors and staff around the Island. I follow it for a bit and watch mothers with babies, an elderly man with a cane, and nurses wearing Crocs and carrying see-through purses step onto the curb at their respective stops.

I separate from the bus and turn left off the main road to find my office. The road hugs the East River until I come to a "T." I'm supposed to turn south there, but instead I sit at the stop sign and stare. Along the shore, the waves lap against the rocks and shrubs, carrying with them a family of ducks out for a lazy morning swim. They seem oblivious to the activities of the Island.

Just beyond the ducks, I see two more islands, islands I didn't even know existed. The southern one is small, with only a few trees and some barren beach. That island's big brother looks much more interesting. It's heavily wooded, and I can just see the tops of a colony of red brick buildings. Squinting to see more, I realize that the buildings are in disrepair and likely abandoned. I learn later that North Brother Island was the home of Typhoid Mary and a host of other unfortunates struck with communicable diseases. *That must have once been a beautiful place to live.*

A loud horn behind me brings me back to reality. I lurch ahead and turn left.

The sea breeze hits me as soon as I get out of the car, and I hear the jingle of the flag line hitting the top of its pole. The seagulls cry and squawk overhead while a mama cat and her kitten scurry past me. I wonder if the birds are warning me to turn back, to return to the safety and freedom of the mainland. *This is not a place for you*, I imagine them saying.

I look up at the gulls and smile. They can squawk at me all they want. I know that I am meant to be here.

ACKNOWLEDGMENTS

The experiences and narratives relayed in this book were many years in the making. I am fortunate to have had supervisors and attending physicians who gave me the freedom to think independently and critically, and advocate for the mission with which I fell in love so early on. Those supervisors, as well as the colleagues, clinical staff, DOC officers, mentors, therapists, and friends with whom I have had the genuine pleasure to work and learn from over those years have all influenced my sense of who I am and who I can be as a psychiatrist. I am deeply indebted to all of them.

I am also grateful and lucky to have been introduced, quite randomly, as it turns out, to several people without whom this book and the personal healing that the writing process produced would not have happened. Michael and Beth Norman, award-winning authors, NYU professors, and husband and wife, took me under their supportive wing in 2010 and taught me about everything from active voice and grammar—things I had lost during my education as a doctor—to maintaining a strong marriage. I have benefited beyond words from their mentorship and friendship.

A serendipitous Christmas Eve meeting in my office at Bellevue in 2013 with a brilliant entrepreneur and now friend, Melissa Thompson, about video psychiatry between the hospital and the jail, led to an introduction to Judith Regan, my publisher. I am still not clear about how Judith ended up at that meeting, but she contacted me very soon after and asked about my interest in writing a book. Not a "tell-all," she was quick to point out, but something that would illuminate the professional world in which I live for an audience that may only know what they read in the papers. I took several months to consider the offer and the impact such an endeavor would have on my family and my professional life. In the end, it was in part Judith's clear sensitivity about the topic and willingness to let me grow and evolve in the writing process that convinced me to take the risk.

I am thankful beyond words that my editors, initially Michael Szczerban and, for the majority of the book, Alexis Gargagliano, provided the freedom, safety, and support for me to write about this system in a way that reflects what I hope comes across as a deep connection with and love for the work. Alexis helped me find a narrative thread in the midst of all of my jumbled writing and has gently guided me throughout this process of self-discovery. The writing and editing, while humbling and arduous, were powerfully therapeutic. I was able to silently record feelings and emotions that I was unable to express in my busy home life with two young children. Through the writing I was able to discover again the joy, curiosity, and inspiration that I experience with patients. Thank you, Alexis.

My family was incredibly supportive during the years of frequently gut-wrenching and pain-staking work on this book and the events that led to its writing. My husband weathered many emotional storms with me and was there on the other side when I emerged. He has felt the strongest impact of the work I do and has steadfastly both respected the space I need and reminded me, sometimes gently and sometimes in moments of complete frustration, to stay connected. His love is powerful and inspiring and has held me together countless times. Honey, thank you. And to my two children, my greatest sources of joy, wonder, and all-consuming love in this world, thank you for giving me the pleasure and honor of being your mom. When I see the world through your eyes, everything good seems possible.

Most importantly, this book would not exist without the patients. I am deeply humbled by their honesty, resilience, and courage, and am indebted to them for the trust they placed in me. In them I see strength and promise instead of sickness and failure. To my patients, I am the most grateful. I hope that this book helps others know you as I have had the privilege to do.